Shape Up!

Shape Up!

A PROGRAM FOR SHIPBOARD PHYSICAL FITNESS

Donald P. Loren
Lieutenant, U.S. Navy

Naval Institute Press · Annapolis, Maryland

Library of Congress Catalog Card No. 79-88437
ISBN 0-87021-626-0

Printed in the United States of America

To my wife Leslie

Foreword

Shipboard physical fitness is an important concern in the navy today. The advent of sophisticated ships and weapons systems, combined with greater personnel technical competency and training, does not lessen the need for today's sailor to be physically fit.

The author and contributing authors have effectively shown the relationship between fitness and overall health, productivity, and attitude. They have presented concepts of physical fitness and diet in terms easily understood and familiar to all navy men and women. Particularly important is the discussion of individual and command responsibilities toward shipboard physical fitness. This text also offers some interesting suggestions on fitness-oriented activities that can be a valuable source of conditioning and recreation at sea.

Shape Up! A Program for Shipboard Physical Fitness is unique in its stress on the importance of physical fitness, diet, and recreation as related to the naval environment. Conscientiously applied, the concepts presented here should benefit both the individual and the navy.

T. B. HAYWARD
Admiral, U.S. Navy
President, U.S. Naval Institute

Preface

On almost any afternoon, the casual visitor to any high school or college can see playing fields filled with young people participating in every type of physical fitness activity imaginable. The Naval Academy, NROTC, or OCS midshipman, as well as the Naval Training Center recruit, are all indoctrinated in the importance of physical fitness. A familiarity with exercise is taught in American educational institutions, creating an environment of healthy, active persons.

Graduation from the training command finds the newly commissioned officer and the new apprentice seaman abruptly removed from a physically active life and thrust into an atmosphere of limited physical fitness activity. The destroyer sailor may find that he is too busy to work out during the day, or that instead of a quick exercise period he needs that extra hour of sleep before he stands the 2000 to 2400 watch. Those persons who desire to continue some sort of conditioning program, and are willing to make the time to exercise, may be thwarted by a lack of facilities or equipment. Long hours, hard work, and a general withdrawal from physical conditioning can completely reverse the life style of staying fit taught during adolescense.

This withdrawal from physical fitness is beginning to generate serious concern within the navy. Health, attitude, and effectiveness are all contingent upon physical fitness. It is important that naval personnel understand the need for remaining fit. Complicating this problem is the limited availability of information concerning shipboard physical fitness for seagoing personnel.

The mission of this book is fourfold. First, naval personnel should be made aware of the need for physical fitness. Second, an understanding of physical fitness should be presented to reflect the concepts of fatigue, exercise, diet, and conditioning. Third, the shipboard sailor should have available a source of exercise programs that can be performed without equipment, onboard a small combatant, in an office, stateroom, or berthing compartment. Finally, supervisory personnel should be familiar with the command and division requirements for maintaining physical fitness, and with the procedure for organizing, officiating, and training participants in a shipboard "smoker."

The author wishes to thank those persons who have contributed to this book in a sincere attempt to bring this subject to the attention of shipboard personnel. Associate Professor Emerson Smith, Head Boxing Coach, U.S. Naval Academy, supplied the basic text for the boxing section. George T. Welsh, U.S. Naval Academy Head Football Coach graciously contributed his ideas concerning warm-up exercises. Dr. Robert L. Slevin of Towson State University kindly provided an outline from which the physical fitness concepts section was written. Lieutenant (junior grade) "Buz" Borries, Ensign Tom Miller, and MM2 Mark Fauber demonstrated the exercises contained in Chapter 4. PH2 Robert Mathis, ET2 Carol Glass, and OS2 Ralph Stevens provided the professional photographs describing each exercise. All of these fine people graciously agreed that royalties from the publishing of this text would be distributed between Navy Relief and the U.S. Naval Academy Memorial Fund.

Chapters 2 through 5 were written by Coach Emerson Smith, Head Boxing Coach at the U.S. Naval Academy. During World

War II, Coach Smith was a Chief Specialist (A) under the Gene Tunney program. While in this program, Coach Smith toured the South Pacific, boxed exhibitions with the middleweight champion of the world, and staged boxing shows in rest and recuperation areas for the U.S. Navy. He has assisted and worked with such notables of the boxing world as Fred Apostoli, Steve Belloise, George Abrams, Freddie Red Cochran, and Anton Christoforidus. Coach Smith is in his twenty-third year as boxing coach at the Naval Academy.

Contents

Shape Up!

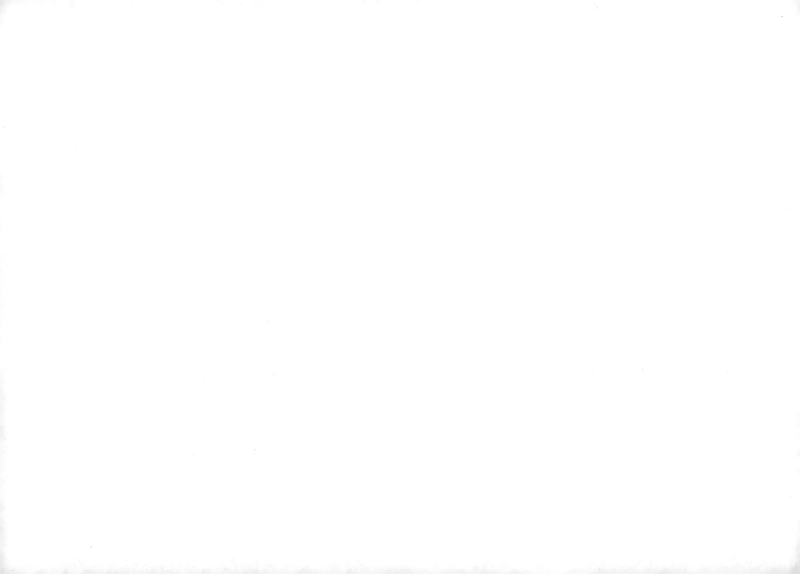

1. Why is Physical Fitness Important to Naval Personnel?

Personal responsibilities toward fitness. The sophistication of a modern, technically oriented naval service is upon us. Sailors no longer climb rigging to unfurl sheets of cream-colored canvas, but instead sit at complex control panels and watch as nuclear fission propels our ships through the water. Passing ammunition is a thing of the past. Today's gunner's mate sits in the combat information center while 5-inch projectiles issue rapidly from an unmanned gun mount. Computers, machines, and elaborate instruments do all the work. The mess deck keeps the crew well fed, and the geedunk supplements the mess should a particular meal not conform to an individual's taste. Surely, it appears that life at sea is considerably less demanding than it was years ago and that today's sailor need not concern himself with being physically fit in order to meet this demand.

If you believe the preceding statement, you have never been to sea. You have never: been a member of a working party loading stores; fired any type of large caliber gun other than a MK 45; worked aloft; worked in an engine room on a stream-driven ship; stood port-and-starboard watches or four hours on and eight hours off for a six-month deployment; tended a mooring line; worked on machinery; swabbed, scowered, or holystoned; manned a fire hose; run the length of a ship setting material condition behind you; crawled beneath a main engine; loaded an anti-submarine rocket; or carried revision three of that letter from the type commander from the captain's office through the chain of command for chop.

Physical fitness is as vital in today's navy as it was seventy-five years ago. The shipboard sailor (this includes the khaki-clad model as well as the blue-denim version) must be physically fit in order to do his job, survive the rigors of life at sea, and to have sufficient energy remaining to enjoy his liberty time ashore (remember liberty time means playing with your kids at the end of the day as well as enjoying that beer in Olongapo). Each individual has a responsibility to himself and to his shipmates to ensure that he is physically able to do his job. Additionally, each of us is responsible to ourselves and our families for maintaining a healthy, energetic, and physically sound condition.

Physical fitness is a state of mind as well as body. It is a determining factor in our overall health, attitude, and even character. The fit person gets more out of life. He does his job better, and enjoys himself more at leisure. He is less susceptible to fatigue, illness, or minor aches and pains, and has the self-satisfying reward of looking fit and trim.

The division/command's responsibilities toward fitness. The various individuals in the navy shipboard community come from many diversified life styles. Some of these people may have developed physical activity as a normal part of their lives, while others may never have been exposed to physical fitness prior to entering boot camp. The command and the division have the responsibility of promoting the concept of physical fitness to all of the people subject to their supervision.

Two vital facets of the shipboard environment are performance of duties and morale. Each of these areas is dependent upon the physical status of the persons composing the organization. The sailor who is always tired, sluggish, overweight, and generally unfit cannot perform his duties adequately. Normal evolutions that require long periods of standing, climbing ladders, moving equipment, and overall endurance cannot be accomplished readily. This slow, half-hearted response can be evidenced in normal work details, watch standing, and shipboard maintenance.

In addition to ineffectual performance, unfit personnel lack vitality and enthusiasm and can develop serious morale problems. The long, hard hours indigenous to a ship at sea can drain a person of all vitality and enthusiasm if that person is physically unprepared for this type of life style. Shipboard physical fitness can be a prime step toward remedying these work deficiencies and morale problems. After working a normal at-sea or in-port day, the physically fit sailor will find himself with sufficient remaining energy for recreation or liberty.

The command has ultimate responsibility for the accomplishment of the ship's mission and for the morale of the ship's compliment. Providing the means for physical conditioning programs and recreational athletic events is an important move toward ensuring that the crew is able to perform capably and enthusiastically. If possible, the recreation committee or the athletic officer could provide a gear issue program so that the ship's company may draw softball, basketball, boxing, and other sporting equipment. The command could also initiate shipboard "smokers," which are an excellent means of establishing physical conditioning, promoting recreational activity, providing interdivision competition, and drawing the entire crew's interest and participation. Any available space may be made into a ship's gymnasium with a few mats and whatever gym gear the ship can purchase.

The division officer plays a very important role in promoting shipboard physical fitness. He must be observant of which people are out of shape or overweight and suggest their participation in a physical fitness program. He should ensure that his people are getting sufficient meals and enough time to eat. A division softball game, basketball game, or bowling match is a fine way to boost morale and provide a means of physical conditioning when the ship is berthed. The division officer can encourage unit participation in ship-organized smokers by "talking up" the event, arranging watch bills to allow contestants time for training and participation, giving support to the division's representatives in the event, and promoting a competitive spirit within the division.

Division officers have additional responsibilities for shipboard fitness. If the command does decide to hold a smoker on board, or chooses to set up an onboard gym space, chances are that one of the division officers will be assigned the collateral duty of executing the plans. The junior officer should be able to set up the smoker, gather competent officials, and train the contestants. He should know what types of fitness programs can be instituted on board ship and how they can be implemented.

The division officer is the driving force behind any physical fitness program instituted by the command. He must be promoter, official, trainer, coach, and cheerleader all in one. His input to the recreation committee and to his division are a vital part of establishing and maintaining a fitness program geared toward developing a fit and spirited ship's company.

2. The Components of Physical Fitness

Modern man is faced with many obstacles that place great strain on his physical fitness and well-being. Such obstacles include quick pace of living, habitual physical inactivity, mechanization, hypertension, coronary disease, obesity, lung cancer, emphysema, bronchitis, and emotional fatigue. Any one or combination of these syndromes of today's society can seriously hinder an individual's "total fitness." Total fitness can be described as:

. . . that state which characterizes the degree to which a person is able to function efficiently. Fitness is an individual matter. It implies the ability of each person to live most effectively within his potentialities. Ability to function depends upon the physical, mental, emotional, social, and moral components of fitness, all of which are mutually interdependent.[1]

Using the concept of total fitness as a foundation, physical fitness is then perhaps best defined by accomplished exercise physiologist H. Harrison Clarke as "the ability to carry out daily tasks with vigor and alertness, without undue fatigue, and with ample energy to enjoy leisure time pursuits and to meet unforseen emergencies."[2]

Certainly, every individual should desire to improve his total fitness and physical fitness posture, yet few people fully understand the concepts of fitness and exercise. The most logical way to examine this topic is to discuss the different types of physical fitness.

There are three types of fitness: passive fitness; muscular fitness; and endurance fitness.[3] Passive fitness is merely that the individual is able to breathe and function without the hindrance of illness or infirmity. Passive fitness is eroded by lack of exercise, which leads the body toward eventual susceptibility to disease. Muscular fitness describes body tone, flexibility, and agility. It is the type of physical fitness that is probably most well known and most commonly developed. Endurance fitness encompasses the continued response of large muscle groups, the functioning of the circulatory system, and efficient operation of the cardiovascular system. The development of endurance fitness is the key to physical fitness and the total fitness concept.

Physical fitness (the combination of passive, muscular, and endurance fitness) is predicated upon ten basic components:[4]

Static (isometric) strength—the ability to exert a maximum force continuously over a brief period of time.

Dynamic strength—the ability to repeatedly exert a muscular force with a consequent progressive decrement in the force that can be exerted.

Dynamic muscular endurance—the ability to execute identical repetitions of a movement over a designated distance in an unlimited amount of time.

Timed static muscular endurance—the ability to execute one continuous muscle contraction (rather than a series of repetitions) for a specified period.

Agility—the ability to rapidly change body position and direction in a precise manner.

Static balance—the ability to maintain body equilibrium in a stationary position.

Dynamic balance—the ability to maintain body equilibrium while in motion or experiencing vigorous movement.

Flexibility—the ability to move the body through as wide a range of motions as possible without undue strain.

Anaerobic power—the ability to exercise for periods of short duration with little dependence on the body's ability to supply oxygen.

Aerobic power—the ability of the body to supply adequate oxygen in order to sustain moderate, continuous work or exercise.

Each of these components, although specific in its own context, contributes to the overall performance of the body in work, recreation, and relaxation. Proper emphasis on developing these areas will result in a fitness program that benefits the entire body and promotes the total fitness concept. Further examination will show how and why each component of physical fitness relates to everyday exercise needs.

Static strength is necessary in performing functions such as lifting, pulling, holding, or pushing. Isometric exercises develop static strength. These exercises consist of actions that require specific muscle groups to exert maximum force for a short duration. Eventual development occurs as the muscle group applies the force longer or applies a gradually increased force each time the exercise is repeated. Some development in muscle tone may be observed, but the primary result of this type of exercising is increased strength of the muscle group (legs, arms, or upper body).

Isotonic or dynamic strength exercises consist of those exercises with which most people are familiar. These include repetitive movements such as push-ups, sit-ups, and weight training. An isotonic exercise causes the actual breakdown of muscle fiber, paving the way for redevelopment of the muscle tissue. This eventual rebuilding results in a newer, more firm muscle with greater definition. The overall effect of the dynamic strength exercise is to produce a trimmer, better defined body.

Dynamic muscular endurance and timed static muscular endurance describe the length of time that the body can support isotonic or isometric activity. Exercises developing these areas increase the period over which the body can exert a pushing or lifting force, and increase the ability to engage in continuous vigorous activity. Lengthening the amount of time over which an isometric contraction is maintained, or progressively increasing the number of repetitions of an isotonic exercise, accomplishes this development.

Agility, static balance, dynamic balance, and flexibility are all measures of coordination. Exercises developing these areas are of extreme importance to athletes, who depend upon smooth body functioning through a wide range of motion. Athletes, of course, are not the only people requiring balance, agility, or flexibility. Everyone needs to develop a reasonable degree of coordination in order to carry out the actions of everyday life. The flexible person is less prone to the injuries, aches, and pains associated with performing routine work. Agility exercises keep an individual energetic and quick. The nonathlete can appreciate the need for agility if he must avoid a fall or other accident.

Aerobic and anaerobic exercises have recently become the

subject of frequent discussion. The physical improvements attained through exercise cannot occur if oxygen-rich blood does not circulate through the body. Aerobic exercises are unsurpassed in their ability to strengthen the circulatory and respiratory systems. Most of our daily lives include some form of aerobic activity; running, climbing, walking, and swimming all employ aerobic principles. Exercises that improve aerobic fitness result in increased overall endurance and a general feeling of invigoration. In contrast, anaerobic exercises do not tax the circulatory or respiratory systems; most isometric exercises fall in this category. Anaerobic exercises serve their purpose in exercising specific muscle groups, but it should be understood that for the development of the entire body as a properly functioning unit, aerobic exercises are essential.

In this chapter, an attempt has been made to explain some of the basics of physical fitness. An understanding of the different components of physical fitness is necessary to the realization of overall fitness requirements and to the establishment of realistic goals for specific areas of development.

3. Diet and Physical Fitness

A total fitness program could not possibly be complete without the correct balance of exercise and proper diet. The body requires a daily intake of nutrients that serve as the fuel for the building materials of life. Certain nutrients are immediately used to repair or produce muscle tissue, while those remaining are stored as fat. Combining the correct intake of these substances with a controlled conditioning plan can result in a trim and firmly toned body.

Food digested supplies protein for growth, nutrients for energy, and vitamins for the formation of enzymes, which act as catalysts in the energy conversion process. The "fuel" that supplies energy for every action of the body is measured in units called calories. The average person may consume as many as 3,500 calories per day. Each process performed by the body requires the use of energy, resulting in the "burn-up" of some of the calories. Those calories not used by the body immediately are stored as fat. If the intake of calories exceeds their use, the body continues to build up layers of excess fat, placing an extra burden on the heart, respiratory system, and muscles because of the increased weight gain. Uncontrolled weight gain is not only hazardous to health, but is also unsightly, demoralizing, and a cause of discomfort and fatigue. Persons who help themselves to a daily geedunk snack will be surprised to learn that eating only twenty-five excess calories per day results in a 2-pound weight gain within a year; consider being 20 pounds overweight in 10 years!

Exercising regularly accomplishes several functions with regard to body nutrition. It increases the flow of blood thus carrying more food and oxygen to the muscles, causes production of new muscle tissue, and results in the burn-up of stored calories. Because different activities burn up varying amounts of calories, an individual's daily routine of work and recreation activities determines how many calories he needs each day and how much exercise is required to burn off excess calories. The following chart depicts caloric expenditure for various activities.[5]

Activity	Calories expended per hour
Standing, sitting	15–20
Reading, writing, eating	80–100
Walking slowly, moving about, sweeping, scrubbing	100–160
Routine shipboard activity	170–240
Heavy work	250–350
Exercising, swimming, engaging in any athletic activity	350–1,000
Running	1,300

Naturally, exercise alone will not reduce the buildup of excess fatty tissue, but as long as caloric intake is kept within reasonable limits, the body that is exercised regularly will be free of unneeded layers of excess stored fat.

The understanding of the basic process of caloric use and storage provides a convincing argument for dietary control, but the shipboard sailor can retaliate with some strong opposing statements. For instance, a ship at sea cannot possibly offer the most complete variety of foods to choose from. Shipboard personnel may ask, "How can I control a balanced diet when the general or wardroom mess decides what I will eat?" or "If I don't eat what is served, I just don't get to eat." There is no question of the validity of these statements, yet their impact on health and diet can be controlled with some extra effort by the individual interested in his own physical conditioning.

Because chow goes down only three times a day, it is advisable to eat at these times and avoid having to satisfy hunger with non-nourishing geedunk meals. Eating a full, balanced meal assures the proper intake of necessary proteins, amino acids, fats, carbohydrates, vitamins, and minerals without the need for any kind of nutritional supplements. Skipping meals in an effort to diet or reduce excess weight is not generally a good idea, because the body requires a daily supply of ruffage for digestion, protein for development, and sugars for energy. A starvation diet, while reducing caloric intake, fails to supply the daily essential nourishment each person needs. Occasionally missing a meal is acceptable if you are not particularly hungry, or if you have something else to do at meal time, but abstinence is not the key to proper diet. (While addressing the topic of when to eat, it should be mentioned that a fourth meal such as mid-rats or an occasional snack is fine as long as it is consumed in moderation and is compensated for by reducing intake at other meals.

The shipboard mess will do its best to prepare the kinds of foods that offer your body the types of nutrients it needs, but it is up to you to ensure that you include these foods in your daily diet. Be certain to eat foods from each of the following four nutritional groups:

milk and cheese
meat, poultry, fish, and eggs
vegetables and fruits
bread and cereals

There are, of course, certain foods to be avoided or at least eaten in moderation. Because of preparation and storage limitations, messing afloat is often characterized by some of these less recommended foods. High calorie and starch-containing foods such as potatoes, gravies, and breads appear often on the weekly mess menu. Limit your intake of these foods to small amounts and do not take seconds. Specific foods to moderate consumption of include:

fat on meats
cooking fats
salad oils
fried foods
gravies and sauces
nuts
pastries
cake
cookies
candies
sugar-sweetened beverages

It is important to briefly discuss what is exactly meant by limiting consumption of a particular type of foodstuff. Foods from the preceding list contain substances such as carbohydrates, fats, sugars, and cholesterol, which can adversely affect your health if eaten in unlimited quantities. They can be responsible for weight gain and deposits of fatty material in the circulatory system (commonly called hardening of the arteries). If these foods are offered on the menu, be sure to take only small portions, or if such a food is offered several times during one week, replace that item with something else. Navy ships are famous for sneaking mashed potatoes, hashed brown potatoes, snowflake potatoes, and French fried potatoes easily onto one weekly menu. Instead of eating potatoes for a fourth time in three days, try taking a larger portion of something else. Raw celery, carrots, salads, and fruits, all usually served at least once a day onboard ship, make excellent substitutes. Eggs can be another oft repeated item, as they are usually served every morning. Try pancakes, French toast, or cereal occasionally and you will reduce your cholesterol and albumin intake appreciably. Please note, however, that your body does need fat, carbohydrates, and cholesterol. Do not make the mistake of completely removing these substances from your diet and by no means should you limit yourself to the variety of sugar-free, salt-free, fat-free, low-cholesterol, or polyunsaturated foods that have flooded today's market. These foods are for people who have been ordered by their physicians onto specific diets.

As you can see, planning your diet requires some serious thought and self-control. Caloric intake should be based upon several factors: First, and most determining, are physical and metabolic considerations. This is sort of a hit-or-miss area, which can best be estimated by experience and needs. Second is a reasonable limitation placed upon consumption of the less desirable substances, as mentioned earlier in this chapter. Third is a consideration for the amount of calories you burn up during normal activity, which can be estimated from the chart in this chapter. The final factor is the very crux of this text; the amount of exercise necessary to burn up extra calories, promote buildup of muscle tissue, and provide an overall healthy and fit feeling.

The remainder of this chapter contains a list of various foods common to shipboard mess deck and wardroom menus, and their caloric values per normal size portion.[6] Using this list, you can estimate and control the number of calories you consume and the number you burn up or need to burn up.

Type of Food	Serving	Number of Calories
MILK AND CHEESE		
Fluid milk		
whole	8 oz.	165
evaporated	4 oz.	170
condensed	4 oz.	490
Cheese		
American cheddar	1 oz.	115
blue cheese	1 oz.	105
cottage cheese	1 oz.	25
cream cheese	1 oz.	105
Swiss cheese	1 oz.	105
Milk beverages		
cocoa	1 cup	235
chocolate milk	1 cup	190

Type of Food	Serving	Number of Calories	Type of Food	Serving	Number of Calories
malted milk	1 cup	280	sausage	2 oz.	135
chocolate milkshake	12 oz.	520	frankfurter	1	155

MEAT, POULTRY, FISH, EGGS, AND NUTS

Chicken					
broiled	3 oz.	185			
fried	2½ oz.	215			

Beef

Type of Food	Serving	Number of Calories	Type of Food	Serving	Number of Calories
pot roast with fat	3 oz.	245	**Fish**		
without fat	2½ oz.	140	fish sticks (5 sticks)	4 oz.	200
oven roast with fat	3 oz.	390	haddock, fried	3 oz.	135
without fat	2 oz.	120	sardines, in oil	3 oz.	180
steak, broiled with fat	3 oz.	330	shrimp	3 oz.	110
without fat	2 oz.	115	tuna, canned	3 oz.	170
hamburger	3 oz.	245	**Eggs**		
corned beef hash	3 oz.	120	fried	1 egg	100
chipped beef	2 oz.	115	hard or soft boiled	1 egg	80
meat loaf	2 oz.	115	scrambled or omelet	1 egg	110
beef stew	½ cup	90	poached	1 egg	80
chili con carne	½ cup	170	**Nuts**		
veal cutlet	3 oz.	185	almonds	15	105
Pork			brazil	5	115
pork chop with fat	2½ oz.	260	cashews	5	95
without fat	2 oz.	130	coconut	2 tbsp.	45
roast pork loin with fat	3 oz.	310	peanuts	2 tbsp.	105
without fat	2½ oz.	175	peanut butter	1 tbsp.	90
cured ham with fat	3 oz.	290	pecans	6	90
without fat	2½ oz.	125	walnuts	6	100
bacon	2 slices	95			

Type of Food	Serving	Number of Calories	Type of Food	Serving	Number of Calories
VEGETABLES			radishes	4	10
asparagus	½ cup	20	sauerkraut	½ cup	15
baked beans	½ cup	165	spinach	½ cup	10
lima beans	½ cup	75	squash	½ cup	50
green beans	½ cup	15	sweet potatoes	½ cup	120
beets	½ cup	35	raw tomatoes	1	30
broccoli	½ cup	20	cooked tomatoes	½ cup	25
brussels sprouts	½ cup	30	tomato juice	½ cup	25
cooked cabbage	½ cup	20	turnips	½ cup	20
coleslaw	½ cup	50			
cauliflower	½ cup	15	**FRUITS**		
celery	2 stalks	10	apples	1	70
corn on the cob	1 ear	65	apple juice	½ cup	60
corn kernels	½ cup	85	applesauce	½ cup	90
cucumbers	6 slices	5	apricots	½ cup	45
lettuce	2 leaves	5	bananas	1	85
raw onions	1 tbsp.	5	blackberries	½ cup	40
cooked onions	½ cup	40	blueberries	½ cup	45
peas	½ cup	60	raspberries	½ cup	35
peppers	1	15	strawberries	½ cup	30
baked or boiled potatoes	1	90	cantaloupe	½ melon	40
potato chips	10 chips	110	cherries	½ cup	30
french fried potatoes	10 fries	155	cranberry sauce	1 tbsp.	30
hash brown potatoes	½ cup	235	cranberry juice	½ cup	70
mashed potatoes	½ cup	115	dates	½ cup	250
pan fried potatoes	½ cup	240	figs	½ cup	90

Type of Food	Serving	Number of Calories	Type of Food	Serving	Number of Calories
fruit cocktail	$\frac{1}{2}$ cup	100	white	1 slice	60
raw grapefruit	$\frac{1}{2}$	50	whole wheat	1 slice	55
canned grapefruit	$\frac{1}{2}$ cup	35	biscuit	1	130
grapefruit juice	$\frac{1}{2}$ cup	60	graham crackers	4 small	55
grapes	1 bunch	45	saltines	2 crackers	35
grape juice	$\frac{1}{2}$ cup	75	doughnuts	1	135
honeydew melon	1 wedge	50	muffins	1	135
lemon juice	$\frac{1}{2}$ cup	30	pancakes	1	60
lemonade	$\frac{1}{2}$ cup	55	pizza	1 slice	180
oranges	1	70	pretzels	5 small	20
orange juice	$\frac{1}{2}$ cup	60	plain rolls	1	115
peaches, fresh	1	35	hard rolls	1	160
canned peaches	$\frac{1}{2}$ cup	100	sweet rolls	1	135
pears, fresh	1	100	waffles	1	240
canned pears	$\frac{1}{2}$ cup	100			
pineapple	$\frac{1}{2}$ cup	35	**Cereal**		
canned pineapple	$\frac{1}{2}$ cup	100	bran flakes	1 oz.	85
pineapple juice	$\frac{1}{2}$ cup	60	corn, puffed	1 oz.	110
plums	1	30	corn flakes	1 oz.	110
prunes	2 tbsp.	150	corn grits	$\frac{3}{4}$ cup	90
prune juice	$\frac{1}{2}$ cup	85	macaroni	$\frac{3}{4}$ cup	115
raisins	$\frac{1}{2}$ cup	230	macaroni and cheese	$\frac{1}{2}$ cup	240
watermelon	1 wedge	120	noodles	$\frac{3}{4}$ cup	150
			oatmeal	1 oz.	110
BREAD AND CEREALS			rice, cooked	$\frac{3}{4}$ cup	150
Bread			rice flakes	1 cup	115
rye	1 slice	55	rice, puffed	1 cup	55

Type of Food	Serving	Number of Calories	Type of Food	Serving	Number of Calories
spaghetti	¾ cup	115	chocolate syrup	1 tbsp.	40
spaghetti with meat	¾ cup	215	honey	1 tbsp.	60
spaghetti with sauce	¾ cup	160	pancake syrup	1 tbsp.	55
wheat, puffed	1 oz.	100	jelly	1 tbsp.	50
wheat, shredded	1 oz.	100			
wheat flakes	1 oz.	100			
wheat flour	¾ cup	300			

FATS, OILS, AND RELATED PRODUCTS

			SOUPS		
butter or margarine	1 tbsp.	100	bean	1 cup	190
salad oil	1 tbsp.	50	beef	1 cup	100

			bouillon	1 cup	10

Salad dressing

			chicken	1 cup	75
french	1 tbsp.	60	clam chowder	1 cup	85
blue cheese	1 tbsp.	90	cream	1 cup	200
mayonnaise	1 tbsp.	110	noodle	1 cup	115
thousand island	1 tbsp.	75	oyster	1 cup	200
			tomato	1 cup	90
			vegetable	1 cup	80

SUGAR, SWEETS, AND RELATED PRODUCTS

			DESSERTS		
caramels	1 oz.	120	angel food cake	2 oz.	110
chocolate bar	1 oz.	145	chocolate cake	2 oz.	420
fudge	1 oz.	115	fruitcake	2 oz.	105
gumdrops	1 oz.	95	gingerbread	2 oz.	180
hard candy	1 oz.	110	pound cake	2 oz.	130
jellybeans	1 oz.	65	sponge cake	2 oz.	115
marshmallows	1 oz.	90	cookies	1	110
			figbars	1	55

Type of Food	Serving	Number of Calories	Type of Food	Serving	Number of Calories
custard	½ cup	140	catsup	1 tbsp.	15
gelatin	½ cup	80	gravy	2 tbsp.	35
ice cream	3½ oz.	130	cream sauce	½ cup	215
apple pie	2 oz.	330	cheese sauce	½ cup	250
cherry pie	2 oz.	340			
custard pie	2 oz.	265			
lemon meringue pie	2 oz.	300			
mince pie	2 oz.	340			
pumpkin pie	2 oz.	265			
pudding	½ cup	125			
sherbet	½ cup	120			

BEVERAGES

ginger ale, carbonated	8 oz.	80
cola, carbonated	8 oz.	105
low calorie, carbonated	8 oz.	10
coffee or tea	1 cup	0
beer	12 oz.	175
whiskey, gin, rum	1½ oz.	100
wine	3 oz.	80

MISCELLANEOUS

olives	6	40
pickles	1	30
popcorn	1 cup	90
chili sauce	1 tbsp.	15

4. Shipboard Exercises

Introduction. If you have just finished reading the first three chapters of this book, you are probably now asking yourself some very important questions. You might be thinking, "How does all of this physical fitness talk relate to *me?*" or "Sure, physical fitness is important, but how does it have a place here on a U.S. Navy vessel in the middle of the ocean?" Well, if you don't have the midwatch today, keep reading and see if you can be convinced that physical fitness can, and should, be incorporated into *your* shipboard life!

Take a good look at yourself. The average American is about ten pounds overweight. If you are not overweight, you may be proportioned such that it is difficult for your body to carry its weight as it is presently distributed. When carrying those excess pounds, your body must work harder to perform everyday functions. Working harder causes muscle fatigue, which causes the muscles to tighten and prevents blood from circulating properly. The overall result is impaired circulation, aches, and pain. This is the reason that so many people tire so quickly after the smallest amount of physical activity.

Fatigued and weakened neck and shoulder muscles can result in severe pain and even headaches. Because most normal watch-standing stations require us to spend much time on our feet, tight neck, back, and leg muscles can not only be a discomfort, but can limit the ability to perform normal watch evolutions. In the second chapter the relationship has already been examined between fitness and the body's overall effectiveness in performing everyday work and relaxation activities, so if you get "winded" while walking up to the bridge to relieve the watch, or if you see that your division LPO is straining to reach for his coffee cup, *it's time to do something!*

Shipboard spaces do not pose a problem to anyone interested in maintaining a healthy and fit body. In addition to executing a planned program of exercise without the use of any gym equipment, the average officer, CPO, or bluejacket can perform hundreds of daily "exercises" without altering his busy schedule.

As you stand in front of the mirror while shaving or brushing your teeth, did you ever realize that you could be exercising? Just pull your stomach muscles in tight, pinch your buttocks together, and hold this position for eight seconds. When you get dressed, bend and stretch as you put on your clothes. This will increase your flexibility and mobility. If you are talking on the sound-powered phone circuit, repeat the stomach-tightening exercise or attempt to "pull the telephone apart" for eight seconds before hanging up the receiver. If seated at a desk, grab the seat of the chair and push your body up off of the chair while extending your legs perpendicular to your trunk. These are just examples of a few simple "nonexercise" exercises, which you can perform routinely during an average day. They employ the techniques of isometric tension to stress and develop commonly used muscle groups and can be excuted in any shipboard space.

The remainder of this chapter is devoted to providing numerous isometric (pp. 21–29) and isotonic (pp. 30–43) exercises that can be performed by all shipboard personnel. These exercises do not require the use of any equipment and can be executed in a limited space. Observe the guidelines set forth in the next section of this chapter, then choose from the groups of warm-up, isometric, and isotonic exercises in order to prepare a realistic program aimed at keeping you physically fit and active.

Getting ready to exercise. Once you have determined your need for a physical fitness program, it is imperative that you take a moment to sit back and plan an exercise program. Here are a few points to examine while starting out on your course toward personal fitness:

1. Set a goal for yourself. It is much easier to work toward a definite result than to set out aimlessly. Such a goal might be set on a weekly basis. Start by thinking, "This week I will exercise on alternate days for one hour a day," and progress from that point.

2. Get a good medical checkup before starting an exercise program. Military personnel normally have regularly scheduled physical examinations, but if you have not seen the medical officer recently, it is a good idea to get a checkup before starting your program. The ship's doctor can advise you on the exercise and diet program you should follow, based upon your age and physical condition.

3. Observe the diet guidelines in this text in order to provide a balanced exercise-diet program of physical conditioning.

4. Plan your exercise program. The exercises in the rest of this chapter can be divided into two categories. The scientific classifications are: *Isotonic*—exercise combining both lengthening and shortening of muscle groups; and *Isometric*—exercise in which no movement of muscle groups takes place. A more practical definition would group these exercises as those that can be performed anywhere at any time of day, and those that require that a certain portion of the day be devoted strictly to working out.

When planning for a workout period, make a list of the exercises you will perform. Next to each of the exercises, include the number of recommended repetitions per set and then write down the number of sets to be performed. For diversity, choose different exercises or change the order in which you perform them. A sample workout program is included at the end of this chapter.

The daily isometric exercises should also be planned, even though they do not require a specific workout period. One plan might be to perform one isometric exercise each time the telephone rings, or each time you sit down at your desk. Set a goal for the number of exercises you will perform during the day.

5. Make exercise part of your normal routine. Try to exercise at the same time of day each day you do exercise. Suggested time periods include, but are not limited to, early morning before breakfast, late afternoon, or just before turning in for the night. Whether you decide to exercise daily or every other day, get into a routine that will allow you to make physical exercise part of your daily activity.

6. Prepare the area in which you are to exercise. If you are onboard a ship that is fortunate enough to have a universal gym and some exercise mats, this problem is solved for you. If you do not have any of this equipment you must make do. Find a small open area. If you can stand up and lie down in this space you are all set to go. For comfort and to prevent chafing of the skin, place a standard blanket beneath you.

7. Dress properly for an exercise period. Many people work

out in their uniforms or street clothes. This is unhealthy, uncomfortable, and does not promote a meaningful workout period. Before exercising, change into a loose pair of gym shorts, a T-shirt, athletic socks, and a pair of sneakers. You will feel comfortable and be eager to engage in a good, hard workout. (Such dress is required only for a period of isotonic exercise. The daily isometrics can be performed in uniform or civilian clothing. The fact that isotonics require total body movement, increased circulation, and deep, full breathing naturally dictates that different clothing be worn.)

8. Prepare yourself mentally for exercising. Review in your mind the goals you have set for yourself and the program you are executing. Try to remove all distractions from your mind.

9. Warm up correctly. The warm-up period is a very important part of any exercise program. Be familiar with the types of warm-up exercises described in this chapter. Keep in mind the fact that the warm-up is designed to prepare the body for working out. Plan these exercises to progress from bending and stretching to increasing heartbeat and breathing.

10. Perform each exercise deliberately, using maximum effort to execute each movement correctly.

11. Do not overexercise! Perform the number of exercises and repetitions that you can handle with only minimal discomfort, and work toward improvement.

12. Be consistent. Exercise conscientiously. Remember that you are working toward your own physical development. Remember, a good exercise program combined with a proper diet will cause you to feel and look more fit, and will help you to work and play with more stamina.

The warm-up exercise. It is essential to begin a period of exercise with a short but effective warm-up. Warm-up exercises serve three very important functions in any type of fitness program: First, a good warm-up prepares the body for exercise by increasing heartbeat and blood flow, thereby allowing more oxygen to travel the bloodstream to the various muscle groups. Second, preliminary stretching exercises ready the large muscle groups for the extensions they will be subjected to during exercise, thus reducing the possibility of injury. Finally, in the few minutes devoted to warming up, when your heart is beating faster, your lungs are filling with oxygen, and adrenaline is surging throughout your body, you are becoming psychologically prepared to exercise, and increasing the probability that you will enjoy a rewarding exercise period.

There are numerous approaches to the theory of warm-up. Some athletes prefer the more conventional exercises, which quickly raise cardiac frequency. These exercises should be performed with submaximal effort for periods of thirty seconds. Four effective warm-up exercises from this group follow.

RUNNING IN PLACE

Jog in place for one minute, lifting your knees as high as possible.

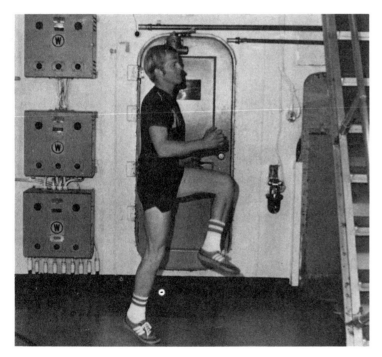

SIDE STRADDLE HOP

Stand erect with feet together and hands at sides. Taking a slight hop, extend legs outward (about two shoulder-widths) and simultaneously raise arms out from sides until they are extended straight up. The exercise is completed by returning to the erect position. Perform these in rapid succession for thirty seconds.

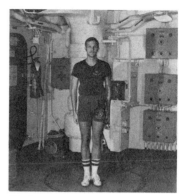

Start

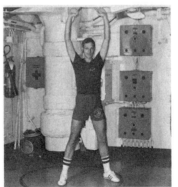

Hop

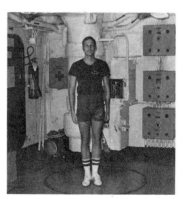

Return

SIX-COUNT BURPEE

Stand erect with feet apart and hands at sides. (Count one) bend to a squatting position with hands on deck next to and outside of feet; (count two) thrust legs back until the body is in the "push-up" position; (count three) lower the body until the chest touches the deck; (count four) push up until the arms are again extended; (count five) return to the squatting position; (count six) return to the erect position. Exercise for thirty seconds, performing rapidly.

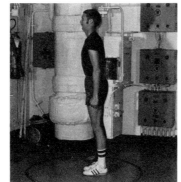
Start

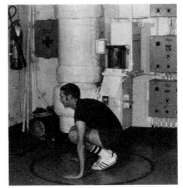
Count One

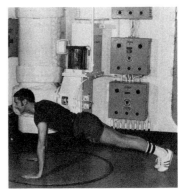
Count Two

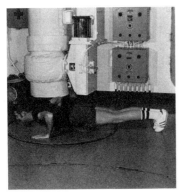
Count Three

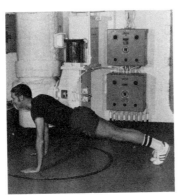
Count Four

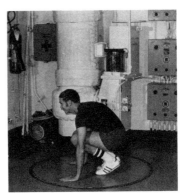
Count Five

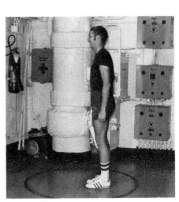
Count Six

18

TOE TOUCH

Stand erect with feet slightly apart and hands at sides. (Count one) raise arms high overhead; (count two) bend at the waist until fingers touch toes; (count three) straighten up with arms still raised; (count four) return to the erect position. Repeat vigorously for thirty seconds.

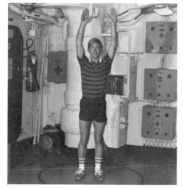

Count One

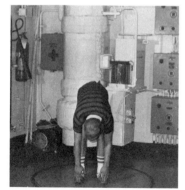

Count Two

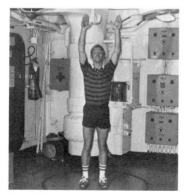

Count Three

A second school of thought concerning warm-up exercises revolves around the concept of flexibility. According to Mr. George T. Welsh, Head Football Coach at the U.S. Naval Academy:

A physically fit person must work for a fuller range of motion in most of his joints. The muscles of the body will stretch and become more flexible if you gradually extend them to a point where you feel some pain, hold for at least eight seconds, relax the muscles, and then try to stretch those same muscles a little further. The muscles must be stretched beyond their normal resting length. "Bouncing" is *not* the way to accomplish this as you do not lengthen muscles unless you hold them in an extended position. When muscles are lengthened by stretching you develop more flexibility in the joints as well as lessen the chances of a pulled muscle when an uncommon strain is placed on those muscles. Full or extreme range of motion will enable you to perform better as well as make you less prone to injury.

The following series of warm-up exercises is the exact routine followed by the Naval Academy midshipmen before a varsity football team workout. Remember to stretch slowly and fully while performing the entire series once.

1. Standing with feet together and knees locked, grasp the back of your calves with your hands and pull your chest down to your knees.

2. Stand with the feet as wide apart as possible, knees locked, and arms folded at the chest. Bend over and try to touch your elbows to the deck. When you can touch the elbows, work to touch your head to the deck.

3. Stand with feet as wide apart as possible with knees locked

and arms out to the sides. Twist your trunk as far to the right as possible, hold, then twist to the left. Keep the upper torso perpendicular to the deck.

4. Stand with feet as wide apart as possible and arms clasped over head. Bend your trunk (do not turn the upper body) as far to the right as possible. Hold, then bend to the left.

5. Stand with feet as wide apart as possible and knees locked. Grasp the inside of each leg and pull your upper torso down as far as you can. Try to touch your head to the deck.

6. While kneeling with legs 4 to 6 inches apart, place your hands at the base of your spine and push forward.

7. Resting on your knees and forearms, spread your knees as wide as possible keeping your feet as wide apart as your knees. Keeping knees and feet spread, raise the upper torso perpendicular to the deck and push the hips forward.

8. Lie on your stomach with your arms out to the sides. Roll your left leg back and try to touch the right hand. Try to keep your shoulders flat on the deck. Hold, then roll the right leg back and touch your left hand. Do not grasp the foot with the hand and pull it up. Work to increase the flexibility in your hips and lower back.

9. Sit with feet together and legs extended. Grasp the right leg below the knee, pull the leg up, and try to touch your chest. Do not bend the knee. Hold, then repeat with the left leg.

10. Sit with feet together and legs extended. Grasp the back of each leg below the knee and pull the upper body down, trying to touch the chest to the upper legs.

11. Sit with the feet as wide apart as possible and knees straight. Touch the deck with both hands directly in front of you extended as far as possible. Relax. Grasp the left toe with both hands (keep legs straight) and try to touch forehead to knee. Relax. Repeat to right toe. Relax. Grasp left toe with left hand, right toe with right hand, and work toward touching your chest to the deck.

12. Sit with knees bent and heels close to the buttocks. Wrap your arms around your shins and rock back and forth on your buttocks, back, and shoulders, and return to the starting position.

13. Lie on your back with arms out to the side. Raise your feet over your head as you roll up on your shoulders, keeping knees straight, and touch your toes to the deck.

14. Lie on your back with the heels as close to the buttocks as possible, and your hands as close to your shoulders as you can get them with the fingers pointing toward your toes. Arch your back, getting up on your hands and toes and raising your stomach as high as you can. Work toward getting the hands and toes close together.

15. From a standing position, extend right leg as far as possible straight ahead into a full split. Point the toes of both feet straight ahead, but as you work to a wider split, roll over on the top of your back foot. Repeat with the left leg forward.

16. Stand erect. Place the right foot in front of the left about 2 feet, pointing the toes straight ahead. Bend the forward knee 90 degrees but keep the left heel on the deck. Place both hands on the hips and push hips forward and shoulders back. Repeat with the left leg forward.

We have looked at two equally valid concepts of warm-up exercise. The shipboard exercise would best benefit from a combination of the two methods. Realizing that the entire scope of this text has been to introduce the seagoing person to the importance of physical fitness, it is evident that the two approaches to warming up, taken separately, will not sufficiently accomplish this goal.

Before your morning shower, start out with the "cardiac" warm-ups. This will wake you up and prepare you for a few minutes of exercise. Follow with several of the flexibility group in order to loosen up and increase range of motion. You are now ready to perform the exercises described in the next section of this chapter.

A combination of the cardiac and the flexibility warm-ups should be used to effect proper preparation for exercise. Vary the combinations as frequently as you would like. Remember, warming up is designed to *prepare* your body for exercise.

DESK SQUEEZE

Purpose. This exercise develops the muscles of the chest (pectoralis) and shoulders (deltoid).

Description. Sit erect, facing your desk. Grasp the sides of the desk and squeeze inward using maximum force for eight seconds. Repeat this exercise while facing away from the desk, reaching behind your back to grasp the edges. Perform this exercise at least ten times during the day.

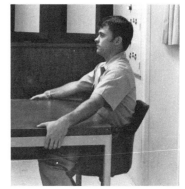

Front

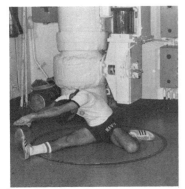
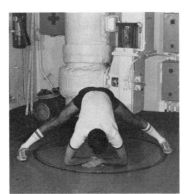

Stretching Exercises

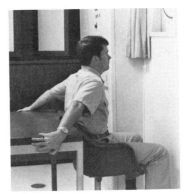

Back

DOORWAY PUSH

Purpose. This exercise develops the muscles of the upper back (trapezius), arms (triceps), and shoulders (deltoid).

Description. Stand in a doorway or narrow passageway and raise your arms until the knuckles touch the door-frame. Tighten your stomach muscles while trying to push the doorway apart. Push using maximum effort for eight seconds, then relax. Perform this exercise at least ten times during the day.

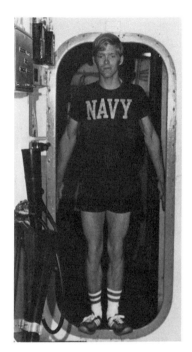

CHAIR PULL

Purpose. This exercise develops the muscles of the shoulders (trapezius and deltoid), arms (triceps, biceps, and flexors), chest (pectoralis), and upper abdomen (rectus abdominis and transversus abdominis).

Description. Sit erect in your chair. Extend your arms straight down and grab the bottom of the seat. Pull up on the seat bottom using maximum effort for eight seconds, then relax. Perform this exercise at least ten times during the day.

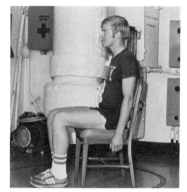

Start

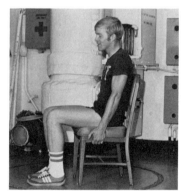

Pull

CHAIR PIKE

Purpose. This exercise develops the muscles of the shoulders (trapezius and deltoid), arms (biceps and triceps), and upper abdomen (rectus abdominis).

Description. Placing your hands on the seat or arms of your chair, raise your feet and legs and hold them perpendicular to your body. Tighten your stomach muscles by pulling them in. Push yourself up off of the chair and hold this position for eight seconds, then slowly lower yourself back onto the chair. NOTE: Keep legs straight and knees locked. Perform this exercise at least ten times during the day.

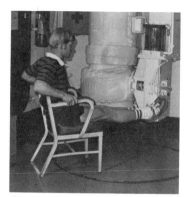

Start

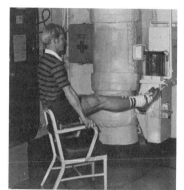

Push

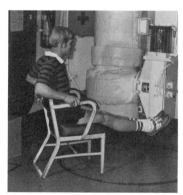

Return

ARM LIFT

Purpose. This exercise develops the muscles of the upper arms (triceps), shoulders (deltoid), and forearms (flexors).

Description. Sit at your desk with your back straight and stomach muscles tight. Raise your arms straight out in front of your body until your knuckles touch the desk. Keeping elbows locked and arms straight, attempt to lift the desk for eight seconds, then relax. Perform this exercise at least ten times during the day.

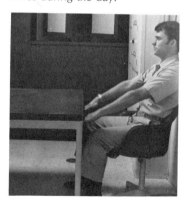

23

BELT CURL

Purpose. This exercise develops the muscles of the upper arms (biceps) and forearms (flexors).

Description. Stand erect with feet shoulder-width apart. Place one end of a belt or towel underneath your right foot and stand firmly on top of it. Grasp the other end with your right hand such that the elbow is slightly bent. Take up any slack in the belt or towel by wrapping it around your hand. Pull upward on the belt using maximum effort for eight seconds, then relax. Repeat using the left arm. Perform this exercise at least ten times during the day.

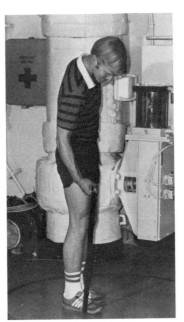

BACK BELT PULL

Purpose. This exercise develops the muscles of the upper back and shoulders (trapezius and deltoid) and upper arms (triceps).

Description. Stand erect, holding belt or towel behind your back, hands approximately 3 feet apart. Keep elbows locked and try to pull the belt apart, simultaneously raising arms upward. Pull using maximum force for eight seconds, then relax. Perform this exercise at least ten times during the day.

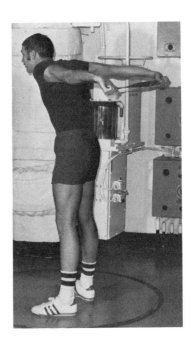

24

FRONT BELT PULL

Purpose. This exercise develops the muscles of the chest (pectoralis) and shoulders (deltoid).

Description. Hold belt so that hands are approximately 3 feet apart. Raise arms in front of body, parallel to the deck, elbows locked. Attempt to pull the belt apart using maximum force for eight seconds. Perform this exercise at least ten times during the day.

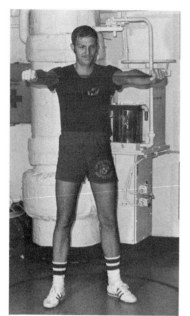

CORNER PUSH

Purpose. This exercise develops the muscles of the upper back and shoulders (trapezius and deltoid) and arms (biceps and triceps).

Description. Stand in the corner of the room facing the corner. Place one hand on each bulkhead at shoulder level (hands should be 6 to 8 inches away from the body). Without moving your feet, push out against the bulkhead using maximum effort for eight seconds, then relax. Repeat this exercise at least ten different times during the day. (This exercise may also be performed while standing in a doorway.)

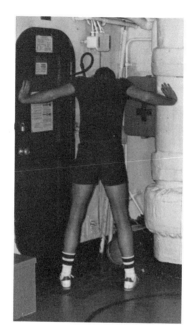

ABDOMINAL TOUGHENER

Purpose. This exercise develops the muscles of the abdominal group (rectus abdominis, transversus abdominis, and internal and external oblique).

Description. When doing routine daily tasks such as talking on the sound-powered phone, shaving, or brushing your teeth, pull in your stomach muscles and hold them tight for eight seconds. Rest for eight seconds, then force the stomach muscles out for eight seconds. The key to this exercise is to associate it with a daily evolution. Hearing the phone ring or growl should remind you to perform this exercise. Do it as many times as possible during the day.

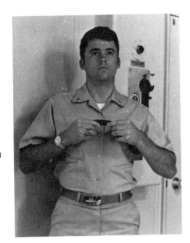

ABDOMINAL SQUEEZE

Purpose. This exercise develops the muscles of the abdominal group (rectus abdominis, transversus abdominis, and internal and external oblique).

Description. Stand with knees slightly bent, feet shoulder-width apart, and lean forward from the waist. Place hands palms down on thighs just above the kneecaps, locking elbows. Inhale, hold breath, contract stomach muscles, and press hands on thighs. Press using maximum force for eight seconds, then relax. Perform this exercise at least ten times during the day.

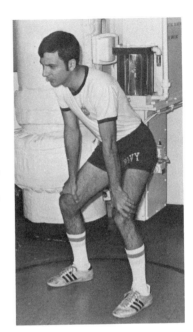

THIGH SQUEEZE

Purpose. This exercise develops the muscles of the chest (pectoralis).

Description. Sit erect with legs shoulder-width apart. Place hands on outside of thighs midway between kneecaps and hips. Push thighs outward while pressing inward with arms. Push with maximum force for eight seconds. Perform this exercise at least ten times during the day.

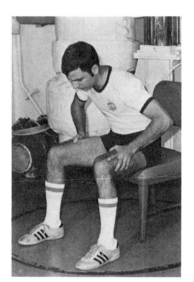

HAND PRESS

Purpose. This exercise develops the muscles of the upper arms (biceps and triceps), shoulders (deltoid), and chest (pectoralis).

Description. Place palms together in front of body at chest level. Raise elbows sideways so that the forearms form a line parallel to the deck. Inhale and press palms together full force for eight seconds. Perform this exercise at least ten times during the day.

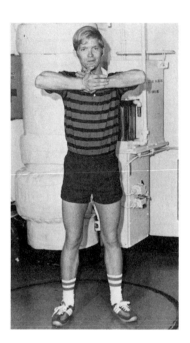

27

ARM FORCE

Purpose. This exercise develops the muscles of the upper arms (biceps and triceps) and shoulders (deltoid).

Description. Stand erect with feet shoulder-width apart. Bend right elbow forward so that right forearm is parallel to the deck at waist level on the right side of the body. Place left hand on top of right hand and press down using full force. Apply pressure for eight seconds, then relax. Repeat with left arm at left side of body. Perform this exercise at least ten times during the day.

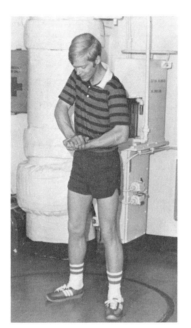

ARM PULL

Purpose. This exercise develops the muscles of the shoulders (trapezius), chest (pectoralis), upper arms (biceps and triceps), and forearms (flexors).

Description. Stand erect with feet shoulder-width apart. Cup hands and interlock by placing one hand on top of the other directly in front of your body. Bend elbows so that forearms are parallel to the deck at chest level. Try to pull hands apart for eight seconds, then relax. Repeat. Perform this exercise at least ten times during the day.

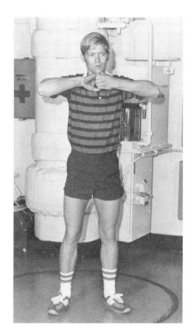

NECK BUILDER

Purpose. This exercise develops the muscles of the neck and upper shoulders (deltoid and splenius capitus).

Description. Stand erect, feet shoulder-width apart, hands clasped behind neck. Push your head backward against resistance of arms, using full force for eight seconds. Repeat this exercise ten times during the day.

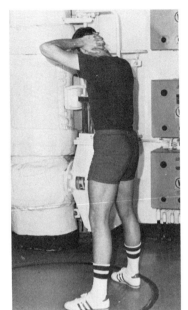

TOE STAND

Purpose. This exercise develops the muscles of the lower legs (gastrocnemius and soleus) and thighs (vastus lateralis).

Description. Stand erect, feet shoulder-width apart. Stand up on the balls of your feet, hold for eight seconds, then return to a normal stance. Perform this exercise at least ten times during the day.

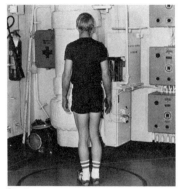

Start

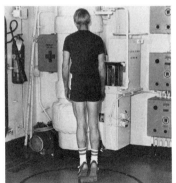

Push-up

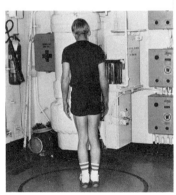

Return

29

LEG LIFT

Purpose. This exercise develops the muscles of the abdominal group (rectus abdominis and transversus abdominis).

Description. Lie supine on the deck and place hands behind neck with fingers interlocked. Keeping feet and knees together, raise feet about 6 inches off the deck and hold for eight seconds, then lower them to the deck and quickly repeat the exercise. Perform in sets of ten repetitions. NOTE: Keep the small of the back flat on the deck (to prevent arching your back). This will effect better development of the abdominal group.

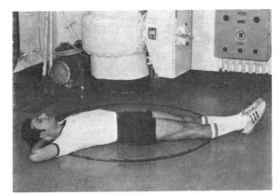

Start

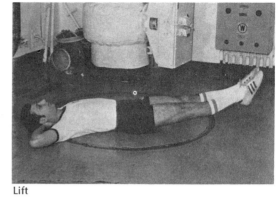

Lift

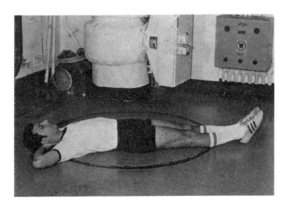

Finish

LEG RAISE

Purpose. This exercise develops the muscles of the abdominal group (rectus abdominis, transversus abdominis, and internal and external oblique).

Description. Lie down on your right side. Lift the left leg as high as possible, then lower it until it almost touches the right leg. Perform this exercise 50 times (working eventually toward 150 times) then turn over and repeat using the right leg. Do not swing your legs up quickly as best results are achieved with moderately slow movement. NOTE: Do not rest by allowing the leg being moved to touch the opposite leg.

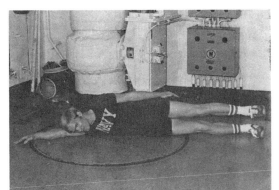

Start

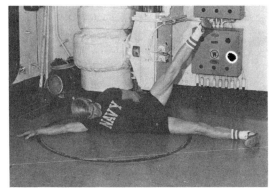

Raise

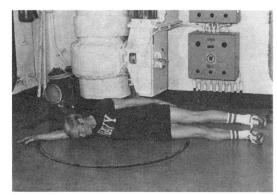

Lower

SIT-UP

Purpose. This exercise develops the muscles of the abdominal group (rectus abdominis, transversus abdominis, and internal and external oblique).

Description. Lie supine on the deck with arms extended behind your head. Inhale deeply and sit up, exhaling as you bend at the waist. Touch fingers to toes, then lower yourself back into the supine position. Perform this exercise in rapid sets of twenty repetitions (start with three sets and work up).

Variation. Perform the same exercise, but this time place your hands behind your neck with fingers interlocked, and bend your knees at a 45-degree angle. When you sit up, try to make your armpits touch the tops of your knees.

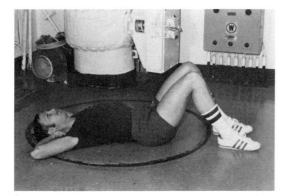

Start

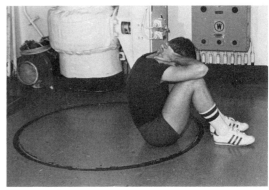

Sit-up

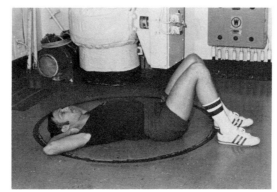

Finish

32

HALF-SIT-UP

Purpose. This exercise develops the muscles of the abdominal group (rectus abdominis, transversus abdominis, and internal and external oblique).

Description. Lie supine on the deck with your feet anchored beneath a desk or locker. Place hands behind your neck with fingers interlocked. Sit up until the upper body is at a 45-degree angle with the deck. Hold this position for eight seconds, then lower your upper body back onto the deck. Perform this exercise in sets of twenty repetitions.

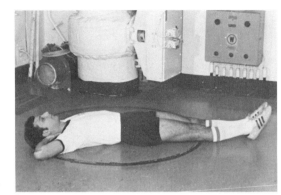

Start

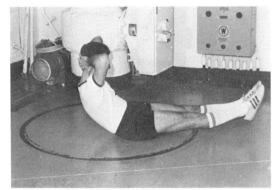

Sit-up

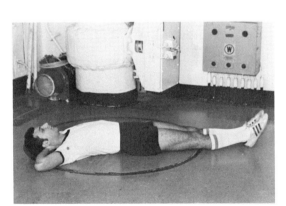

Finish

33

V SIT-UP

Purpose. This exercise develops the muscles of the abdominal group (rectus abdominis, transversus abdominis, and internal and external oblique).

Description. Lie supine on the deck, legs straight, feet together, arms extended straight back overhead. Sit up and simultaneously lift both legs, trying to touch fingers to toes, then lower upper body and legs back onto deck. Perform this exercise in sets of twenty repetitions.

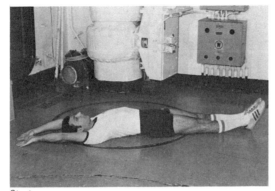
Start

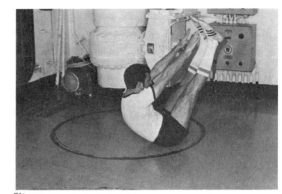
Sit-up

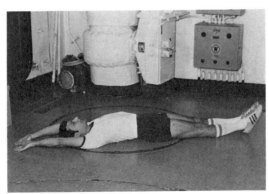
Finish

34

INCLINED SIT-UP

Purpose. This exercise develops the muscles of the abdominal group (rectus abdominis, transversus abdominis, and internal and external oblique), back (latissimus dorsi and teres major), and thighs (vastus lateralis, sartorius, and gluteus maximus).

Description. Sit to one side of an armless chair that is about 3 feet from a desk or locker. Anchor both feet beneath the desk and interlock hands behind neck. Slowly lower upper body until entire body forms a straight line at a 45-degree angle to the deck. Hold this position for eight seconds, then sit up until upper body is again perpendicular to the chair. Perform this exercise in sets of ten repetitions.

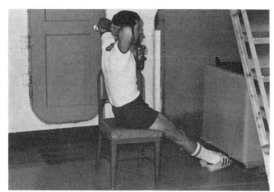

Start

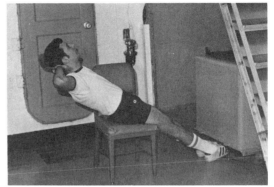

Lower

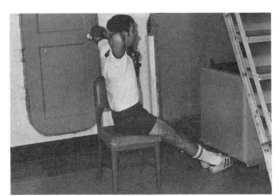

Finish

35

ALTERNATE TOE TOUCH

Purpose. This exercise develops the muscles of the trunk (external and internal oblique and latissimus dorsi).

Description. Stand with feet two shoulder-widths apart and arms straight out from sides, parallel to the deck. (Count one) bend at trunk so that left hand touches right foot; (count two) return to the starting position; (count three) repeat by touching right hand to left foot; (count four) return to the starting position. Perform this exercise in sets of twenty-five repetitions.

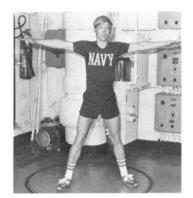
Start

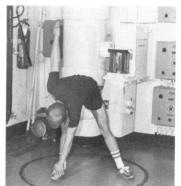
Count One

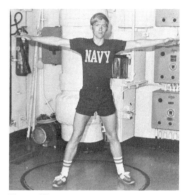
Count Two

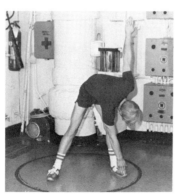
Count Three

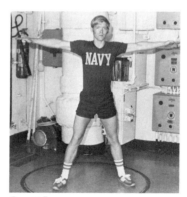
Count Four

FOUR-COUNT TWIST

Purpose. This exercise develops the muscles of the abdominal group (rectus abdominis, external and internal oblique, and transversus abdominis).

Description. Lie supine on the deck with arms outstretched. Raise legs so that they are perpendicular to the body. (Count one) lower legs to the left until they almost touch the deck; (count two) raise them again to the perpendicular position; (count three) lower them to the right; (count four) return to the perpendicular position. Repeat this four-count exercise in sets of ten repetitions. NOTE: Do not let your legs touch the deck. Keep legs straight and knees locked.

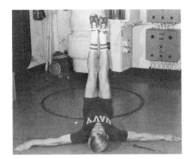

Start

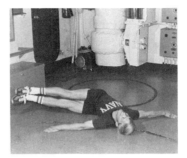

Count One

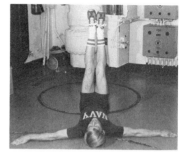

Count Two

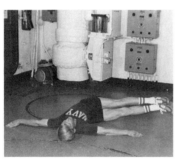

Count Three

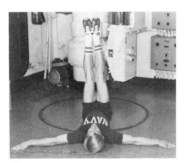

Count Four

STANDING TWIST

Purpose. This exercise develops the muscles of the abdominal group (internal and external oblique).

Description. Stand erect with legs shoulder-width apart. Extend arms outward from sides until parallel with the deck. Twist to the left extending right arm straight forward, perpendicular to the starting position. Then twist to the right extending left arm forward. NOTE: For best results, stretch through full range of motion. Perform this exercise in sets of twenty-five repetitions.

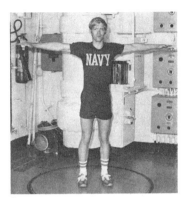

Start

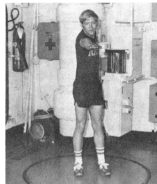

Twist

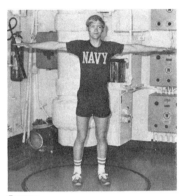

Return

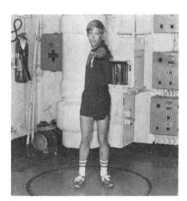

Twist

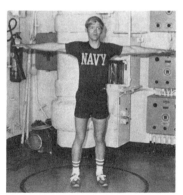

Finish

SEATED TOE TWIST

Purpose. This exercise develops the muscles of the trunk (internal and external oblique), back (latissimus dorsi, serratus anterior, and teres major), and legs (biceps femoris, gastrocnemius, and gracilis).

Description. Sit down on the deck with your legs spread at a 45-degree angle, knees locked and legs straight. Extend arms straight out from sides, perpendicular to your body. Twist your body at the waist so that the right-hand fingers touch the left toes. Twist in the opposite direction so that the left hand touches the right toes. Perform this exercise in sets of twenty-five repetitions.

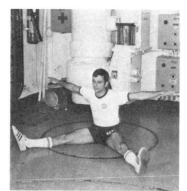
Start

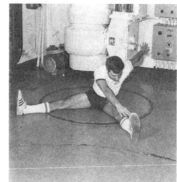
Twist

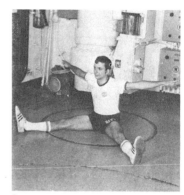
Return

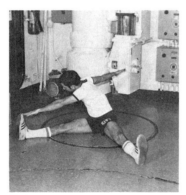
Twist

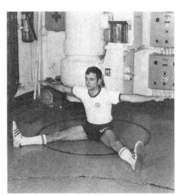
Finish

CHEST STRETCH

Purpose. This exercise develops the muscles of the chest (pectoralis) and shoulders (trapezius and deltoid)

Description. Extend arms straight out in front of body, parallel to the deck. With one sharp motion, thrust your elbows straight back as far as possible, keeping arms parallel to the deck. Return arms to the starting position. Perform this exercise in sets of five repetitions ten times during the day.

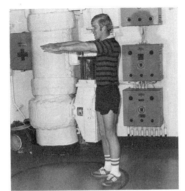

Start

ARM CIRCLES

Purpose. This exercise develops the muscles of the shoulders (deltoid), upper back (trapezius), and chest (pectoralis).

Description. Stand erect with feet shoulder-width apart. Raise arms out from your sides, parallel to the deck. Swing arms forward in circles approximately 2 feet in diameter. Perform twenty-five times, stop, then repeat in the reverse direction.

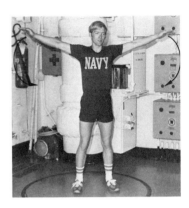

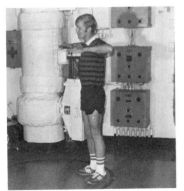

Pull Back

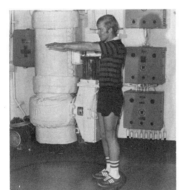

Finish

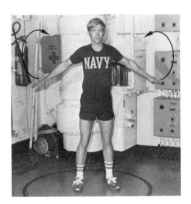

DESK PUSH-UP

Purpose. This exercise develops the muscles of the shoulders (trapezius and deltoid) and chest (pectoralis).

Description. Stand erect about 3 feet away from your desk, stateroom sink, or an anchored chair. Place hands palms down on the desktop edge. While keeping your body straight, slowly lower yourself until your chest touches the edge of the desk. Once in this leaning position, push down on the desk using full force for eight seconds, then slowly push yourself back up until arms are fully extended again. Perform in sets of twenty repetitions.

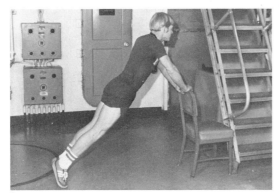

Start

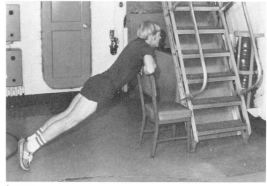

Lower

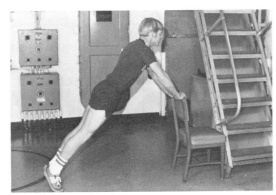

Push Up

PUSH-UP

Purpose. This exercise develops the muscles of the arms (biceps and triceps), shoulders (trapezius and deltoid), and chest (pectoralis).

Description. Lie prone, hands palm down on deck next to body at about midchest. Keeping back straight, push up slowly so that the entire body is supported on your hands and the balls of your feet and arms are fully extended and elbows locked. Then lower your body until your chest barely touches the deck. NOTE: The key to this exercise is keeping your back straight at all times. Perform this exercise in sets of twenty repetitions.

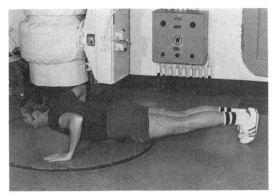
Start

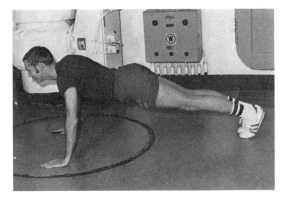
Push Up

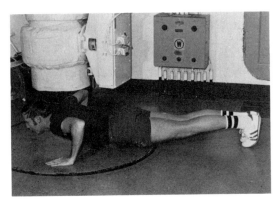
Lower

TREADMILL

Purpose. This exercise develops the muscles of the lower abdomen (rectus abdominis) and legs (rectus femoris, vastus lateralis, sartorius, and gastrocnemius).

Description. Lie prone, hands palm down on the deck next to the body at about midchest. Keeping back straight, push up until elbows are locked and your entire body is supported on your hands and the balls of your feet. This is the starting position. (Count one) move right foot straight foward so that your right knee is tucked in close to your chest; (count two) move right leg back to the starting position; (count three) move left foot forward to the tuck position; (count four) return to the starting position. Perform this exercise in sets of twenty-five repetitions.

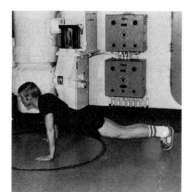

Start

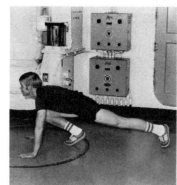

Count One

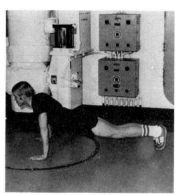

Count Two

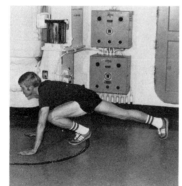

Count Three

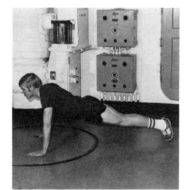

Count Four

43

Sample workout program

Exercise	Repetitions	Sets
Week 1		
WARM-UPS		
Toe touch	20	1
Stretching exercises	NA	NA
Side straddle hop	25	1
Six-count burpee	10	1
Running in place	1 minute	NA
EXERCISES		
Seated toe twist	20	1
Sit-up	20	1
Push-up	20	1
Chest stretch	10	1
Toe stand	10	1
Half-sit-up	20	1
Leg raise	50 each leg	1
Leg lift	10	1
V sit-up	20	1
Standing twist	25	1
Four-count twist	10	1
Inclined sit-up	20	1
Push-up	20	1
Hand press	10	1
Running in place	2 minutes	NA

Exercise	Repetitions	Sets
Week 2		
WARM-UPS		
Toe touch	20	1
Stretching exercises	NA	NA
Side straddle hop	25	1
Six-count burpee	10	1
Running in place	1 minute	NA
EXERCISES		
Seated toe twist	20	1
Sit-up	20	1
Push-up	20	1
Chest stretch	10	1
Toe stand	10	1
Half-sit-up	20	1
Leg raise	55 each leg	1
Leg lift	10	1
V sit-up	20	1
Standing twist	25	1
Four-count twist	10	1
Inclined sit-up	20	1
Push-up	20	1
Hand press	10	1
Belt curl	10	1
Arm force	10	1
Running in place	2 minutes	NA

Exercise	Repetitions	Sets	Exercise	Repetitions	Sets
Week 3			**Week 4**		
WARM-UPS			WARM-UPS		
Toe touch	20	1	Toe touch	20	1
Stretching exercises	NA	NA	Stretching exercises	NA	NA
Side straddle hop	25	1	Side straddle hop	25	1
Six-count burpee	10	1	Six-count burpee	10	1
Running in place	1 minute	NA	Running in place	1 minute	NA
EXERCISES			EXERCISES		
Seated toe twist	20	1	Seated toe twist	20	1
Sit-up	20	1	Sit-up	20	2
Push-up	20	1	Push-up	20	2
Chest stretch	10	1	Chest stretch	10	1
Front belt pull	10	1	Front belt pull	10	1
Back belt pull	10	1	Back belt pull	10	1
Toe stand	10	1	Toe stand	10	2
Half-sit-up	20	1	Half-sit-up	20	1
Leg raise	60 each leg	1	Leg raise	65 each leg	1
Leg lift	10	1	Leg lift	10	1
V sit-up	20	1	V sit-up	20	1
Standing twist	25	1	Standing twist	25	1
Four-count twist	20	1	Jumping rope	2 minutes	1
Inclined sit-up	20	1	Four-count twist	20	1
Push-up	20	1	Inclined sit-up	20	1
Hand press	10	1	Push-up	20	2
Belt curl	10	1	Hand press	10	1
Arm force	10	1	Belt curl	10	2
Running in place	2 minutes	NA	Arm force	10	1

Exercise	Repetitions	Sets	Exercise	Repetitions	Sets
Neck builder	10	1	Four-count twist	20	1
Seated toe twist	20	1	Belt curl	10	1
Running in place	2 minutes	NA	Arm force	10	1
			Hand press	10	1
Week 5			Neck builder	10	1
			Sit-up	20	NA
WARM-UPS			Running in place	2 minutes	
Toe touch	20	1			
Stretching exercises	NA	NA			
Side straddle hop	25	1			
Six-count burpee	10	1			
Running in place	1 minute	NA			

Note: Isometric exercises performed throughout the day should supplement each workout program.

As you progress, add or delete exercises, increase the number of sets, and increase the time for running in place.

Exercise	Repetitions	Sets
EXERCISES		
Seated toe twist	20	1
Standing twist	25	1
Chest stretch	10	1
Push-up	20	2
Sit-up	20	2
Leg lift	10	1
Half-sit-up	20	1
Front belt pull	10	1
Back belt pull	10	1
Toe stand	10	2
Leg raise	70 each leg	1
Push-up	20	2
Sit-up	20	2
Inclined sit-up	20	1

5. A Guide for Boxing Smokers

Introduction. One of the most effective ways of promoting physical conditioning is to incorporate exercise and enjoyable competition. Shipboard life limits the extent of such sporting competition, but there are certain athletic events that can be scheduled depending upon the size of your ship. The most universal of all navy sporting events is the boxing smoker. Little space or equipment is needed and all of the ship's complement is generally eager to participate or observe.

There is, unfortunately, a tendency for shipboard boxing smokers to evolve into great disorganization. Results of a poorly organized program usually include: little physical benefit for the participants; injuries caused by improper training and preparation; and a generally uninteresting slugging match between two exhausted boxers. This is where the division officer comes into play (let's face it, you'll probably be the JO responsible for the event). If you follow some very basic rules about training, preparation, officiating, and technique, your ship's boxing smoker can be a productive and enjoyable event. The next section of this text is a step-by-step set of instructions for organizing a shipboard boxing smoker. Read the eleven following guidelines and keep them in mind as you read further and, later, plan your boxing event.

Boxing smoker guidelines. The following eleven guidelines should be the foundation of any boxing smoker:

1. Emphasize skill. The boxer must be taught to outpoint his opponent. Discourage slugging and rushing and do not permit the trading of punches.
2. It is important for every coach to plan, supervise, and conduct all workouts.
3. Each coach must be aware that certain individuals do not belong in boxing competition. Consideration must be given to the participants' health, attitude, physical and emotional condition, and level of training.
4. Insist on a planned medical supervision program.
5. The *objectives* of the program must be clearly understood. Administrators, officials, participants, and spectators must be made aware of the safety requirements of the program.
6. Accept and purchase only the best protective equipment available (ring, gloves, headgear, deck padding, etc.).
7. Headgear and mouthpieces must be standard equipment.
8. Constantly strive for ways to make the sport injury-free.
9. Work out a systematic way to match all boxers skillwise, in practice and competition.
10. Select and train officials who can quickly recognize when a boxer is hurt, overmatched, or not able to protect himself.
11. Always remember that a boxing smoker is not designed to develop professional boxers. The program is established to provide exercise, relaxation, and a source of spirited shipboard competition.

The administration of a boxing smoker

Selection and duties of officials

The selection of officials must be closely supervised. Of these men, the referee is the one whose competence is of the most importance. The safety and conduct of your boxing matches will depend on the ability of the referee selected.

A. Qualities necessary to a good referee:
1. A complete and thorough knowledge of the rules.
2. The ability to apply the rules during the excitement of the match.
3. Good judgment, common sense, and the courage to uphold his convictions; referees should always bear this in mind: "Render your verdict as you see it."
4. The ability to be in the right place at the right time; to be agile and alert.

B. Uniform:
1. A referee's uniform should be comfortable, distinctive, and at the same time inconspicuous. The latter characteristic is an advantage, because no one attends a boxing smoker to watch the referee. A referee has performed well if the audience and contestants say that they did not notice him.
2. It is recommended that the referee wear:
   a. White shirt.
   b. White or black trousers.
   c. Black bow tie.
   d. Black belt.
   e. Sneakers.

C. Prebout Duties:
1. Arrive and dress early.

2. Visit both coaches and answer their questions, if any, concerning the rules.
3. Confer with the officials.
4. Instruct seconds and contestants.
   a. Emphasize clean breaks.
   b. Demonstrate foul blows.
5. Supervise wrapping of hands.
6. Inspect gloves.
   a. Regulation gloves must not be broken in the region of the knuckles.
   b. Metal ends on laces should be cut off.
7. Inspect bandages.
8. Inspect cups; aluminum, Bakelite, or standard cup protectors should be worn.
9. Inspect the ring; ring should be 18 feet square covered with a 2-inch-thick pad and canvas cover.
10. Have the bout commence on time.

D. Duties in the Ring
1. A good referee can either make or break a shipboard boxing smoker. As each round starts, the referee should glance at each corner to see that the seconds have cleared them of buckets, stools, towels, and other equipment.
2. The ring ropes must be looked upon as sacred. No one, including the referee, should ever be permitted to lean on the ropes or clutter them up with towels, bath robes, or other equipment. Enthusiastic seconds often are great offenders in this respect.

3. In accordance with AAU rules, boxers are required to shake hands at the beginning of the bout. Any contestant who refuses to shake hands may be disqualified by the referee. The touching of both gloves is considered a handshake. Except for shaking hands at the beginning and finish of a contest, no other hand shaking is permitted.
4. The rules do not allow the referee to touch the boxers except under unusual circumstances.
5. A referee should never pass between the two boxers or turn away from them. He is required to keep both boxers in view at all times.
6. The referee should position himself so that he has an inside view of both boxers.
7. It has been found desirable for the referee to keep constantly in motion, generally in the direction of the movement of the competitors, but never faster than the boxers.
8. The referee shall use the following commands.
   a. "Break" when ordering each boxer to step back before boxing.
   b. "Stop" when he wants both boxers to cease boxing.
   c. "Box" when asking boxers to continue.
   d. When two boxers clinch, the referee commands "Break," at which time both boxers are required to take one step backward. Failure to step back calls for a warning. Whenever the referee finds it necessary to issue a warning, he must first say "Stop," making sure that the boxer addressed does not relax his attention on his opponent in order to listen to the referee. It is after such warning that the term "Box" is used to resume the bout, or whenever the match has been stopped.
9. When a boxer is knocked down:
   a. The bout shall not continue until the referee has reached the count of eight.
   b. When a boxer has risen from a knockdown, the referee shall check his gloves for resin or dirt.
   c. The referee should always look at the eyes of a boxer who has been knocked down. If the boxer can look at the referee, has good coordination, and can move and properly defend himself, the bout should be allowed to continue. If the boxer is overmatched or if he cannot focus his eyes, shows unstable motion, and cannot defend himself, the bout should be stopped.
   d. Suspend the count on a knockdown if one of the boxers fails or delays going to a neutral corner.
10. Stop the bout:
    a. If it seems to be too one-sided.
    b. If the contestants are stalling.
    c. To warn a boxer of a rule infraction.
11. Terminate a contest if a contestant has received an injury.
12. The referee should raise the hand of the winner.

THE JUDGE

Judging in boxing is truly a subjective art, and good judges are often tough to come by. The decision of a judge is the expression of his opinion based upon the evidence, which he notes as each round progresses. In most cases, good judges will be unanimous in their decisions. In a tight contest, however, it is not unusual that the judges disagree, because the seating position of one judge might very well give him a completely different look at the blows landed.

The two judges shall be stationed on opposite sides of the ring. It shall be the duty of the judges to watch every phase of the bout and to record their decisions by rounds. The judges shall keep count of the rounds, time-outs, and knockdowns, and, in general, cooperate with the referee. It is important that the judges know the skills and techniques of boxing as well as the rules and the infractions of the rules.

At the end of each contest the two judges and the referee will declare a winner. (You may use three judges instead of using the referee if you prefer. The CO, XO, other senior officer, or someone who is already familiar with boxing rules should be instructed as to judging responsibilities and employed as an official. If you ask these persons to be judges, you not only have impartial officials, but have everyone from the captain on down involved in the shipboard smoker.) Each judge shall add the points allotted to each contestant in the three rounds, and write his decision on the scoring slip.

A. The competent judge:
1. Must be alert.
2. Must be capable of quickly assessing the evidence.
3. Must mentally review the complete round.
4. Must be selfconfident of his ability.
5. Must have a thorough knowledge of the rules.

B. Scoring:
1. Ten points shall be allotted to the winner of each round.
2. The loser in each round shall be allotted any number of points below ten.
3. If the round is even, each boxer receives ten points.
4. No fractions of points may be awarded.
5. Points shall be awarded for the following.
   a. Attack and defense.
   b. Blocking, parrying, and other defensive maneuvers.
   c. Generalship (generalship is rated when the points are otherwise equal). The decision should be in favor of the boxer who displays the best generalship and style. The term "generalship" shall indicate the development of natural advantages, coupled with intuition and the ability to grasp quickly the advantage of any opening given by an opponent.
   d. Aggressiveness. Aggressiveness indicates willingness of the contestant to press the attack with due regard for his own protection.
6. When awarding points observe the following:
   a. Number of hits. Each hit that lands in accordance with the rules shall be awarded a point.
   b. Defense. The successful avoiding of blows such that the attack of the opponent is thwarted shall be considered in awarding points.
   c. Correct hits. Points shall be awarded for direct, clean hits with the knuckle part of the closed glove, on any part of the front or sides of the head, or on any part of the body above the belt. Hits on the arms do not count.

Backhand blows are not permitted.

d. Attacking and tactics shall be considered after each round.
e. Foul blows must not be counted. If the referee warns one of the competitiors for a foul, the judges shall award points to the other boxer.

7. Fouls
a. Each hit below the belt, tripping, kicking, or butting.
b. Hits or blows with the head, shoulder, forearm, or elbow.
c. Throttling of an opponent, pressing with arm or elbow in an opponent's face, and pressing an opponent's head back over the ropes.
d. Hits with the open hand, the inside of the glove, the wrist, or side of the hand.
e. Hits landing on the back of an opponent, especially any blow on the back of the neck or to the kidney.
f. Any attack made while holding on to the ropes or making use of the ropes in any way.
g. Wrestling, lying on top of an opponent, or throwing punches while in a clinch.
h. An attack on an opponent who is knocked down. (Disqualification should be considered appropriate.)
i. Holding an opponent's arms or head while clinching.
j. Holding or pulling an opponent while hitting him.
k. Completely passive defense by means of double cover and intentionally falling to avoid a blow.
l. Useless agressive or offensive utterances during the round.

Sample score card Ten-point system

name	first round	second round	third round	total
Jones (red)	10	10	6	26
Smith (blue)	8	10	10	28
WINNER	Smith	Official		
		(signature)		

Guide for awarding points

description of round	round winner	round loser
Very close	10 points	9 points
Clear advantage demonstrated but no knockdown	10	8 or 7
Round one-sided	10	6 to 4
Boxer outclassed (referee should stop bout)	10	3 or 2
Points indicate round even; (+) indicates better style	10+	10

8. If a boxer has received a foul blow and declares himself unable to continue the bout, the referee shall, if he has seen the foul committed, use his discretion in determining action. If the referee finds that the victim of the foul is unable to continue through no fault of his own, he shall stop the bout, disqualify the opponent and award the decision to the boxer subject to the foul.

9. Decisions. There are four types of decisions:
   a. Win by knockout.
   b. Win by retirement of opponent (i.e., opponent incapacitated).
   c. Win by disqualification of opponent.
   d. Win by decision based on points.

A competitive boxing program has as its prime purpose the outscoring, outthinking, and outmaneuvering of one boxer by another through the medium of well-placed blows and well-executed defensive moves. In order to win by points, a boxer must show superior technical skill, ring strategy, and good physical condition.

THE TIMEKEEPER

The timekeeper is a very important official and should not be appointed merely because he can read a watch. Although the timekeeper functions somewhat as an accurate and dependable machine, it is also his duty to closely cooperate with the referee. He must signal the start and finish of each round, relay the count to the referee, and take time-outs as instructed by the referee.

A. Duties:
   1. The timekeeper must be at ringside close to the bell and buzzer.
   2. He shall ring the bell to start each round.
   3. Ten seconds before each round, the timekeeper shall give warning to the boxers' seconds by sounding the buzzer. (A whistle or a compressed air horn works equally well.)
   4. He shall follow the referee's advice when stopping the bout.
   5. He shall immediately start his knockdown count as soon as the standing boxer steps toward the furthest neutral corner. The count must be loud and clear so that the referee can hear, and shall be "1–2–3–4–5–6–7–8–9–out." The referee will pick up the count when he is satisfied that the opponent has gone to a neutral corner. The referee's is the official count.

B. The length of each round should be adjusted according to the experience level of the contestants and the amount of time spent getting in shape for the event. For inexperienced boxers: three one-minute rounds, each separated by a one-minute rest. For experienced boxers or boxers with one month of preparation: three two-minute rounds, each separated by a one-minute rest.

C. If a boxer is knocked down and gets up before the referee counts "out," but then falls again without having received another blow, the timekeeper continues the counting from the point where he stopped. If both boxers are down together, counting continues as long as one of them is still down. If both boxers remain knocked down until the "out" count is reached, then the bout is stopped and the decision is given based upon the total points awarded up until the time of the knockdown. In the event of a knockdown, the fallen boxer must take a mandatory eight-count.

THE SECOND

The second is to a boxer what a nurse is to a baby. It is the second who must advise the boxer throughout the bout. He should watch every movement of the opponent, learn his shortcomings, and impart this knowledge to his boxer. There should be an outside and an inside second for each corner.

A. Duties of the outside second:
1. Watch time of round.
2. Have stool ready when ten seconds remain in the round.
3. Set stool tightly in corner.
4. Make boxer comfortable, placing his hands on his knees, feet flat, sitting straight and relaxed.
5. Take mouthpiece out and rinse it.
6. Hand water to inside second.
7. Replace mouthpiece at ten-second buzzer.
8. When bell rings, lift boxer off stool.
9. Take gloves and headgear off, wipe down boxer, and place robe on boxer at the end of the bout.
10. Make certain boxer shakes hands with opponent.

B. Duties of the inside second:
1. Put boxer at rest between rounds.
2. Wipe face and body clean.
3. Attend to cuts and bleeding.
4. Check gloves and laces.
5. Give instructions when 10 or 20 seconds remain in the time-out.
6. Analyze opponent and make short, concise suggestions for the next round; the inside second should know all the skills and rules necessary to help his boxer defeat the opponent.
7. Show good sportsmanship and encourage boxer.
8. Be cool, calm, and collected.

THE ANNOUNCER

The announcer announces the names of the judges, timekeeper, medical officer, referee, the weight class of the upcoming bout, and the names of the contestants (mentioning the contestants' hometowns and divisions). He shall collect the score sheets and announce the decision of the judges and referee.

THE BOXERS

The boxers, of course, have the responsibility of providing an exciting and sportsmanlike competition. Here are some rules concerning general technique and ring etiquette.
1. Always box from the on-guard position.
2. Never stop moving.
3. Work with leading side punches.
4. Never throw a single jab.
5. Jab directly from your shoulder and return a jab along the same axis.
6. Protect your chin with your power hand when jabbing.
7. Do not drop your jab.
8. Do not drop your power hand when jabbing.
9. Do not stand in a corner or lean on a ring rope.
10. All defensive moves should include a counter.
11. Mix up offense, defense, and counters.
12. Hit to the body, not to the arms or shoulders.
13. Be relaxed.
14. As soon as the boxers enter the ring they should shake hands and return to their respective corners.
15. When introduced, the boxer should go to the center of the ring and bow quickly in the direction of the judges.

Sample Announcer's Sheet

Fill in for appropriate bout.

Begin announcement in the center of the ring:

"The officials for this evening's bouts are" (pointing as the names are called):

Judging   1. _____

               2. _____

               3. _____

Timekeeper _____

Medical Officer _____

Referee _____

First bout _____

Second bout _____

Third bout _____

Fourth bout _____

(Check and complete for each bout.) Announce each bout as follows.

"In the first bout of the evening, wearing the white jersey, in the blue corner, in the 155-pound class, from _____, repre-
_(hometown)
senting _____ division, weighing _____, _____. In
_(division)   _(weight)   _(boxer's name)
the red corner, wearing the _____, from _____, repre-
_(color jersey)   _(hometown)
senting _____ division, weighing _____, _____."
_(division)   _(weight)   _(boxer's name)

Immediately following the last round, the announcer will enter the ring, collect the slips and announce the decision: "The winner, in the _____ corner, _____."
_(color)   _(winner's name)

16. If the referee corrects the boxer, the boxer must nod and comply—never argue or act upset.
17. At the conclusion of the bout, boxers should return to their respective corners, remove gloves and headgear, and return to the center of the ring when the referee calls.
18. When the decision is announced, boxers should shake hands, politely bow toward the judges, and leave the ring.

Checklist for a boxing smoker

The following is a checklist for use by smoker officials before the event.

1. Number of matches
2. Experience of boxers
3. Prebout meal
4. Headgears
5. Size of gloves (10-, 12-, 14-oz. depending on weight class)
6. Mouthpieces
7. Boxing shoes
8. Boxing protective cups
9. Wrapping hands
10. Medical examinations
11. Resin and resin boxes
12. Microphone
13. Bell
14. Time clock
15. Ring
16. Ten-second buzzer, whistle
17. Water buckets
18. Bottles for corners
19. Judges' stations
20. Ring stools
21. Judges' slips
22. Programs
23. Officials

Instruction of boxing smoker contestants. Obviously, no one can become an experienced boxing coach in a few lessons. However, the fact remains that it is possible to grasp the broader aspects of the subject, which may be combined with fundamental skill already obtained through individual boxing.

All coaches must appreciate that condition is the most important factor in the life of a boxer. He may be as clever as Jim Corbett or hit as hard as Jim Jeffries, but if he lacks condition, all those attributes mean very little.

Coaching is a combination of handling men to the best advantage, imparting skill, and developing a high spirit of competition.

In logical order, coaching begins with the squad and continues through the team to the individual. It also involves the consideration of the opposition and conditions of competition.

Coaching the squad

Preparation for competition begins on the day the squad responds to a call to boxing. Regardless of the number of candidates who respond, the number may decrease considerably soon after work begins. Boxing has strong appeal, but in the cases of some candidates this is soon offset by the work involved.

In contrast to those who first report and then drop out, there will be a small number of potential candidates who for one reason or another do not show up on the first call. Since all participation is voluntary, some coaches operate on the assumption that if a man isn't interested enough to report, he isn't worth following up. However, it is well known that many a meet has been won by a boxer who was first introduced to the sport by members of the squad or through personal contacts by the coach.

Workout procedure

The boxing workout is an individual matter and should be governed by conditions and needs. Each workout should be approached with a sense of purpose. Always work at full speed and stop while still feeling fresh and desiring more. Fatigue causes careless work and, therefore, the formation of bad habits. It is during this time that accidents occur.

A general workout program is as follows.

Round 1—Warm up with shadow boxing.
Round 2—Skip rope.
Round 3—Work on heavy bag.
Round 4—Box.
Round 5—Work on light bag or pulley weights.
Round 6—Do calisthenics.

Four weeks should be allowed for preparation, to train boxers so that they may be able to compete skillfully and without injury. A sample workout plan would be:

1600–1615 Dress for boxing, warm up slowly.
1615–1620 Talk about workout for that day.
1620–1630 Run four two-minute rounds with one-minute rests (conditioning).
1630–1640 Do boxing exercises (conditioning).
1640–1645 Do footwork drills (skill work and conditioning).
1645–1655 Teach the left jab and defenses (skill work or fundamentals).
1655–1700 Put on headgear and gloves and match boxers according to weight and ability.
1700–1715 Put eight men in the ring for corner boxing, one on offense, one on defense. Work on left jab and defenses (skill work and fundamentals).
1715–1720 Do neck and stomach exercises (conditioning).
1720–1730 Run in place or on deck, if appropriate; end of practice (conditioning).

Twenty to thirty workout days of 1½ hours per day should be ample preparation for an excellent boxing smoker.

Coaching the individual

One point of wide contrast between individuals hinges upon the amount of work they are willing to put into practice. One person may believe that even a little effort may exhaust him just before a bout, whereas another will work too hard simply because he has been cast in the role of a workhorse.

Another point of wide difference involves injury. Some men will conceal a bruised hand, whereas others will "baby" it to the extreme. Perhaps there is no single point in boxing calling for better judgment on the part of a coach. In this connection it is advisable to call upon the medical officer for an opinion. To ask a man to box against his will or hold him in check when he feels he is fully qualified for a hard workout is likely to create mistrust and discontent.

Some individuals are highly sensitive and become depressed by defeats even in practice bouts, while others are thick-skinned and rugged. If by any chance a boxer shows signs of avoiding actual contact in the ring, it will become necessary to sit down with him and go over the entire picture.

Some few contestants will work harder for special favor than they will for their own improvement. It should be an unfailing rule, of course, never to allow personal likes and dislikes to creep into any phase of coaching. Many a meet has been lost by mistaking a pleasing personality for ability or by entering a contestant simply because he is the elected captain or highly popular with the squad.

It is not expedient here to give complete details as to diet, training, and similar phases in the shaping up of an individual since this may be worked out on the basis of accumulated experience. In following any standardized routine, it must be remembered that what sometimes is "one man's medicine" is "another man's poison." Only by recognizing this situation can a coach bring his team individuals to a point where the team as a whole will function at greatest skill, courage, and endurance.

The following specialized training activities are essential to the learning of boxing skills and obtaining boxing conditions:

Rope skipping	Calisthenics
Shadow boxing	Road work
Boxing	

Rope skipping

This is a valuable aid in developing stamina, speedy footwork, and the proper use of the feet without undue effort. Instinctive moves of the feet are bettered and perfected by the rhythm and sustained effort of the boxer who uses this exercise.

Rope skipping also limbers up the muscles of the arms, wrists, and shoulders. The light movement makes the muscles supple and responsive to the coordination of mind and leg movements.

When skipping rope one must always be on the toes. Throw the rope forward and, as it passes in front of the body, raise both feet together to allow the rope to pass under them. The hands, holding the handles of the rope, should describe a revolving motion as this is done.

It is easier to learn how to skip rope by lifting both feet in unison. After one has learned forward skipping, he should learn backward skipping by throwing the rope back over the head.

After mastering these two moves, try skipping with one foot in front of the other. Later, try reversing the position of the feet with each turn of the rope.

Many other moves, such as the double jump, loop jump, and kneel, can be learned through practice and patience. All of these help a boxer to shift his feet quickly, gracefully, and automatically.

Shadow boxing

Shadow boxing is the best method of acquiring correct form. It should be used to correct boxing skill. It teaches ring movement, hitting sequence, speed, and relaxation. Each blow should be practiced and perfected before going on to another. While shadow boxing, the boxer should move deliberately in, out, and around, punching hard all the time. The boxer should plan each round before beginning to shadow box.

Boxing

The best way to learn how to box is to box! While boxing, the boxer should work toward some definite objective. One should box with all types of individuals—tall, short, slow, and fast. Timing and judgment of distance can only be developed through actual boxing. One should try to learn something from each man boxed.

Calisthenics

The aspiring boxer must realize that each part of his body must be exercised and strengthened as much as possible. The extension of the arms, the abdominal muscles and the neck muscles should receive special attention.

The arms are used continually. They tire easily unless specially trained. The abdominal region is the "mark" for which all boxers try, and therefore well-developed stomach muscles are essential. The neck must be able to absorb the shock of the head blows.

The following exercises are especially adapted for the boxer:

Sit-up	Leg lift
Leg raise	Push-up

Road work

There is no substitute for road work. It is the only form of exercise that gives one the stamina and durability needed to carry on the tireless pace boxing calls for.

Road work strengthens the heart, lungs, and legs. The heart will be able to adjust to the strenuous exertion. The lungs will be better able to supply more oxygen and the legs will be better able to support the body during a bout.

Since shipboard confinement prohibits actual road work, running in place or doing several laps around the flight deck will have to suffice. Breathe deeply and evenly and do not go to extremes by running until exhausted. Use good judgment, and when you think you have had enough, call it a day. It is best to maintain a steady pace to your road runs. Pay attention to your breathing. By doing so you will be able to carry on longer with less effort to your breathing apparatus. Never run too soon after a meal. At least four hours should elapse between eating and strenuous exercise.

Ring generalship

This is the art of using boxing skills and tactics. The boxer must think and act under extreme pressure. Pace, style, counters, and defensive skills become the tools of the boxer's trade. Ring generalship then is the ability to take advantage of the opponent's weaknesses and also the ability to keep the opponent's strength to a minimum.

HOW TO BOX THE INTERNATIONAL JABBER

1. Move, use the whole ring and lots of lateral moves.
2. Use your left or right jab counters.
3. Use head and shoulder moves and work on infighting.
4. Look for mistakes of dropped lead and counter with power hand and hooks or jabs.

HOW TO BOX THE OPPOSITE STANCE

1. Lead with power hand while moving to power. Come back with lead hand, with jab or hook.
2. Circle away from power jab and cross and move laterally.
3. Use a double power hand to head and body.

HOW TO BOX THE TALL OPPONENT

1. Use the whole ring.
2. Be aggressive with low head and shoulder moves, and be aggressive when inside position is obtained.
3. Hit with combinations and move.

SCOUTING THE OPPONENT

Scout your opponents as much as possible. Look for and record both their strong and weak points. Do not put out information that will make your opponent mad. Try to use sparring partners that box like the opponents.

Basic boxing skills

The on-guard position

The on-guard position is the basic boxing stance from which all of the offensive and defensive moves are initiated. While in this position, the boxer should have his muscles in a relaxed tone. He should only apply muscle tension when delivering a blow or making a quick defensive move.

The basic on-guard position:

1. The left foot is forward and at a 40-degree angle, pointed inward. The left food is flat and the knee is loose. The left leg and left side of the body should form a straight line. The body weight is now primarily on the left leg. The right foot is back, pointed forward. The knee is slightly bent with the heel raised.
2. The trunk is basically controlled by the position of the left leg. In the proper position the left side of the body is forward, exposing a narrow target. A more aggressive fighter may want to square his body to aid in his attack. However, for defensive purposes the narrower target is more effective.
3. The left arm should be forward with the elbow pointed toward the deck. The hand should be at shoulder height about 8 to 10 inches from the shoulder. The forearm should be relaxed and hinged at the elbow. Forearm tension should not be needed to hold hand in position.
4. The right arm should be in close to the body, with the elbow pointed toward the deck. The hand should be forward and in

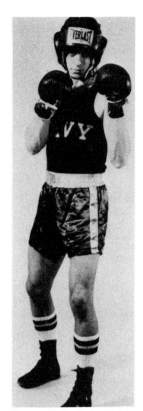 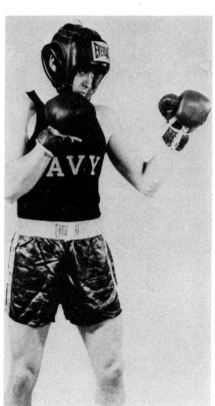 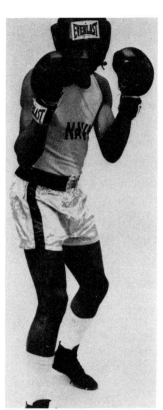 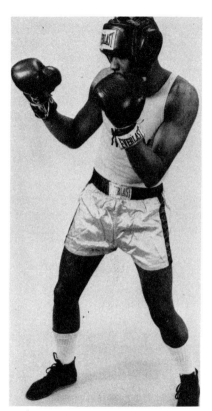

On-guard Position, Right-
handed Stance

Side View

On-guard Position, Left-
handed Stance

Side View

line with the left shoulder. The hand should be held open with the palm toward the opponent. The arm should be hinged at the elbow with the forearm relaxed.

5. The vision should be focused on the chest area of the opponent. This will help the boxer to react to and anticipate the start of an opponent's blow.
6. The headgear is worn so the eyebrows are completely covered. The top and chin straps should be snug on the head so the headgear will not turn or slip off.

Hitting

Before attempting to strike an opponent, the boxer must know the proper way to make a tight fist. The fingers should be in the center of the palm and the thumb should be across the second and third fingers.

When a blow is delivered it should be straight and accurate. The reason for using the straight punches is because they are safer, easier, and quicker. The hand should be twisted as the arm is being extended so when contact is made the knuckles are up. The arm should return quickly to the on-guard position. The hips should be loose and allowed to swing freely. This will increase the power of the punch.

A hook or a swing should be used minimally because it leaves the body exposed and vulnerable to attack. One must remember that defense and safety should be emphasized in this program.

Fundamental blows

There are seven fundamental blows:

the jab
the cross
the hook to the head
the hook to the body
the jab to the body
the cross to the body
the uppercut

The jab may be used as a power punch or just to ward off an opponent. The punch begins with pushing off of the right foot and shuffling the left foot forward. The left hand strikes out hard to the extended position, driving hard to the chin, nose, and forehead. The hand should be twisted with the knuckles up on contact.

The cross is a power punch. It begins with the shift of the body weight to the left side. The rear foot should pivot forward to aid the hip and shoulder turn on the right side. At the same time, the right arm hand is rotated upward and is driven forward toward the opponent's chin. On contact the knuckles should be up and the palm down.

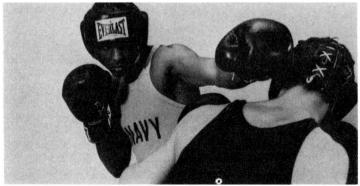

Jab to the Head

60

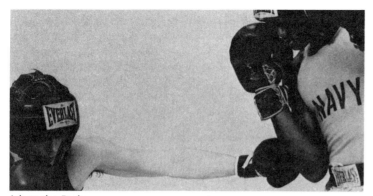

Jab to the Body

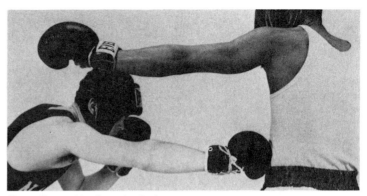

Cross (Power Hand) to the Body

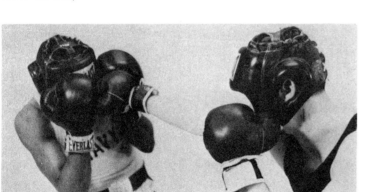

Cross (Power Hand) to the Head

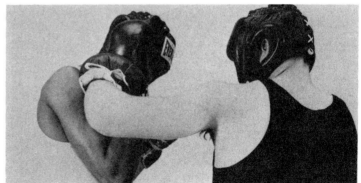

Hook to the Head

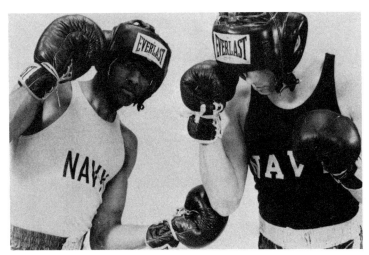

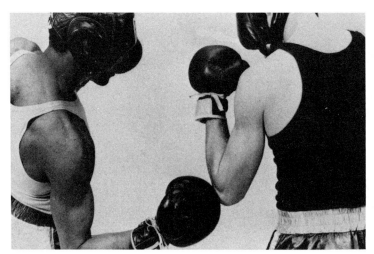

Hook to the Body

Uppercut

The jab to the body and cross to the body are basically the same punches as the jab and the cross, respectively. The differences come from the fact that the boxer is crouched and the blow is delivered to the body. In order for the blow to be effective the boxer should be on the same level as the intended point of contact.

The more advanced types of blows that may be effective if executed properly are the bent arm blows. These are the hooks and the uppercuts.

The hooks may be divided into the hook to the head and the hook to the body. These blows carry the full force of the body behind them and are used primarily for infighting. The movements of the body are reversed for the right and left hands.

The left hook to the head begins with a twist of the left hip and shoulder to the centerline of the body. The weight is shifted to the right leg and the left arm is whipped in a tight circle at head level. On contact, the palm of the hand is pointed inward with the thumb-side up.

The left hook to the body is basically the same blow as the hook to the head. The variation is manifested in the height of the shoulders. The left hand should remain at shoulder height to keep the boxer from telegraphing the punch. The legs are bent to lower the point of impact of the punch. On contact the palm should be inward and the thumb-side of the hand should be up.

The uppercut begins with the body bent forward and to the left side. The forearm is parallel to the deck. The shoulders and hips begin to twist to the centerline as the hand comes up. The elbow should remain bent and the fist should cross in front of the body. On contact the palm should be upward. A good uppercut should strike the opponent in the solar plexus.

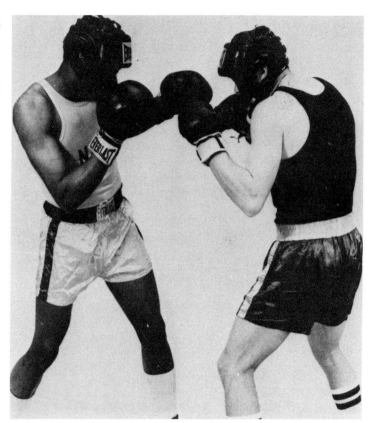

In-distance

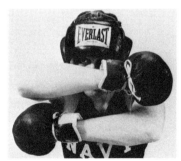

Cover Position

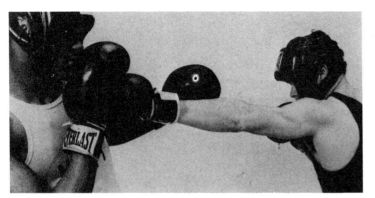

Parrying the Jab

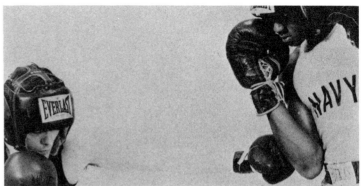

Blocking the Jab to the Body

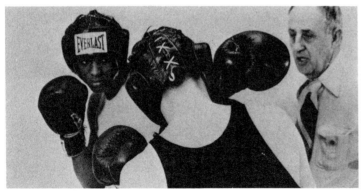

Sliding the Jab

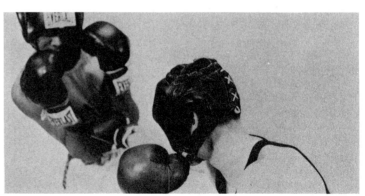

Blocking the Cross (Power Hand) to the Body

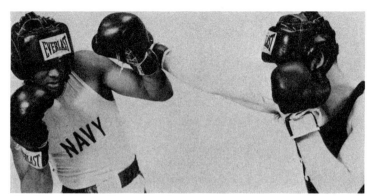

Blocking the Cross (Power Hand)

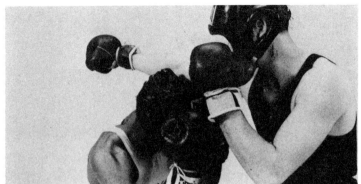

Ducking the Cross

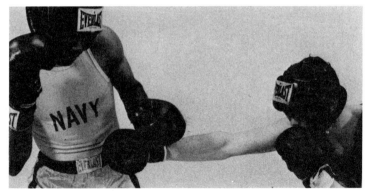

Drop-parrying the Cross

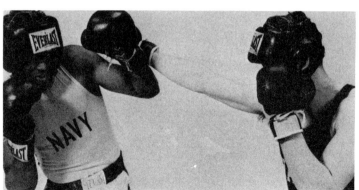

Body Roll and Forearm Block Against the Cross

Fundamental blocks

A. Catch—catch on-coming blows in palm of glove.
   1. Right-hander versus right-hander—catch blow in palm of right hand.
   2. Right-hander versus left-hander—catch blow in palm of left hand.
   3. Left-hander versus left-hander—catch blow in palm of right hand.
B. Parry—deflect on-coming blow with partially open defensive hand.
   1. Right-hander versus right-hander—parry blow with palm of right hand.
   2. Right-hander versus left-hander—parry blow with palm of right hand.
   3. Left-hander versus left-hander—parry blow with palm of right hand.
   4. Left-hander versus right-hander—parry blow with palm of right hand.
C. Slip—move head and shoulders to right to avoid blow.
D. Snap away—move backward quickly, just far enough to make opponent miss. The chin should be kept down and the hands high and close to the head.
E. Forearm and elbow blocks—involves the movement of the left arm (up, down, or sideways). It is effective against punches to the body.
F. Cover-up—the gloves are in front of the face, but positioned so the boxer can see between them. The arms are forward and covering the body. The elbows are in tight and pointed toward the deck.

Fundamental footwork

There are only four possible moves involved with footwork: advance, retreat, circle left, and circle right.

There are many variations to these basic movements, and they will come naturally once the boxer has learned the basic movements.

Forward Shuffle—the body position is maintained at all times. The foot movements are no more than 2 inches in length, the left foot leading, followed by the right. Both feet should be on the floor at all times.

Backward Shuffle—the same as the forward shuffle except the right foot leads the left.

Quick Advance—a long step forward toward the opponent. The left foot moves first, followed by the right.

Quick Retreat—a long step backward involving a shift in the weight to a stiff right leg. The left foot should follow the right.

Circle Left—the left foot moves first, followed by the body wheeling to the fundamental position.

Circle Right—the left foot moves to the right from 4 to 6 inches, followed by the right foot.

The hands should be coordinated with the movement of the feet at all times. The left lead should be used when the left foot is moved, the right when the right foot is moved. When circling left, the boxer should be ready for his opponent's right counter. When circling right, the boxer should be ready for his opponent's left hook.

Aggressive defensive drills and counters

These drills are designed to increase the aggressiveness of the defensive fighter. They consist of defenses and counters.
1. Offensive jab, defensive parry, and counter jabs
2. Offensive jab, defensive parry, and counter cross and hook to head
3. Offensive jab, defensive slip inside and counter hook to body, hook to head, cross to head
4. Offensive jab, defensive duck, and counter cross to body, hook to head, cross to head
5. Offensive cross, defensive shoulder roll, and counter cross, hook to head
6. Offensive cross, defensive head and shoulder move backward, and counter cross, hook to head
7. Offensive hook, defensive forearm block, and counter hook to head

NOTE: These drills are both offensive and defensive. It is essential to execute them correctly, both in offense and defense. Work hard on improving form and quickness instead of power.

Sparring techniques
1. Select a man of your size and ability.
2. Select good headgear and a good set of gloves. Use vaseline on face, gloves, and headgear. Wear a rubber mouthpiece.
3. Work on quickness, form, and quick short combinations. Do not run in; work to maintain the proper foot position.
4. Hit and move. Snap away and use lateral moves. Do not stop, ever. If you do stop you should cover, duck, and move laterally.
5. Spar to outpoint your opponents. The best method is by using the jab.
6. Work from the front side; the jabs are the safest leads—use them.
7. Learn to relax and box the full time: two-, three-, or four-minute rounds.
8. Be aggressive with your defense. Aggressiveness with defense means the ability to handle punches that include counters.
9. Be aggressive with your offense; stress quickness and lightning-fast combinations. You must deliver punches without getting hit.
10. Always protect your head; move, cover, jab, maintain body rhythm, head and shoulder moves, and duck movements.
11. Sparring is an art. The class boxer is the man who can work and box with anyone. To do this you must have skill and ability. Boxers who have command of the skills can make any sparring partner look good, while displaying class himself.

First aid hints for handling boxing injuries

It should be evident that some boxing injuries are inevitable, as in all contact sports. When a boxing injury does occur, it is important to be able to estimate just how serious the accident is. The corpsman and doctor should be called as quickly as possible when injuries seem to be of serious nature.

Fracture—A fracture is a broken bone. The injured person will feel a snap at the base of the injury. Roughness or bone irregularity will be felt over the fracture. Tenderness or sharp pain will be present with the slightest movement. If you suspect a fracture refer to a doctor or corpsman. *Do not move the injured person.*

Fractured Jaw—Pain on movement of lower jaw or irregularity of teeth will be evident. Do not move the jaw. Take the boxer to the doctor.

Fractured Nose—The nose, if broken, will usually bleed profusely. The nose will be swollen and deformed. Refer to doctor.

Concussion—The most common head injury in boxing is concussion. In case of a knockout, avoid unnecessary handling. *Keep the man warm* and call a doctor or corpsman. *Let the man remain on the deck and remove his mouthpiece.*

Definitions of terms used in boxing

blocking	Rendering an opponent's blow ineffective by blocking it with the hands, shoulders, or arms.
breaking	Stepping back from a clinch.
clinching	Holding an opponent so that he is unable to make an attack.
corner boxing	Technique used to learn in-distance offensive and defensive skills. Protection is afforded by ring floor padding and ring ropes. Excellent way to learn fundamentals and to accommodate large numbers of men.
counter	Return of a blow.
covering	Holding arms in front of face and body to prevent the opponent from getting a clean shot at the vulnerable spots of the body.
cross counter	Slipping a blow and countering.
crouching	Bending at the waist to deliver or avoid a blow.
drawing	Drawing body backwards to avoid a blow.
feinting	Any action intended to mislead the opponent into thinking that an attack is about to be made.
footwork	The movement of the feet to enable the boxer to maintain poise and to help him adapt to all phases of defensive and offensive boxing.
foul blow	Hitting below the belt, hitting in clinches, or any other move that is not legal.
head and shoulder moves	Moves that keep the head a moving target.
hook	Striking from the side with a short curved motion of the arm.
infighting	Boxing at close range.

jab	Fast straight blow with lead hand.
lead	Taking the initiative in attacking an opponent.
one-two punch	Simultaneous delivery of two blows, namely, left and right cross.
one-two-three punch	Simultaneous delivery of three blows, namely, left jab, right cross, and left hook.
on-guard	In a position to deliver a blow or guard against a blow.
parrying	Diverting an opponent's blow by striking the attacking punch with the palm of the hand.
shadow boxing	Boxing with an imaginary opponent, performing with snap and precision all moves used in actual contact work.
sliding roll	Technique used to move under punches and to counter to body.
slipping	Moving the head to either side to avoid a blow.
southpaw	A left-handed fighter, one who punches with strong or power left hand or jabs with strong right.
uppercut	Upward motion of the arm with the palm turned in toward the target.

Boxing ring construction. The boxing ring for a shipboard smoker does not have to be an elaborate edifice to the glory of

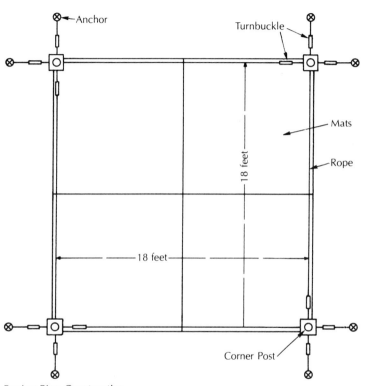

Boxing Ring Construction

69

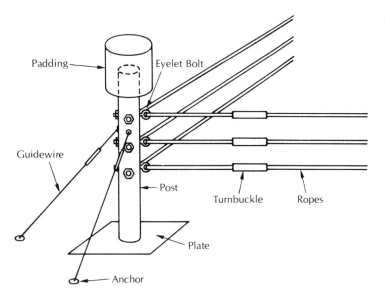

Padding

Eyelet Bolt

Guidewire

Post

Turnbuckle   Ropes

Plate

Anchor

small stuff and canvas wrapping. Manila line will suffice if wire rope is not available.

The ring ropes can be attached to the corner posts by common eyelet bolts. The first rope should be fastened 4 feet from the bottom of the post. The second and third ropes are then spaced at 3 feet and 2 feet from the bottom. Splice a turnbuckle into each length of rope so that any slack may be taken up and tension may be applied to the ropes.

Anchor the corner posts by attaching two guide wires $3\frac{1}{2}$ feet from the bottom of each post. The guide wires should be perpendicular to each other. Splice a turnbuckle in each of the guide wires in order to take up any slack. Fasten the guide wires to any bulkhead or deck hardware (the aircraft hold-down hardware on the flight deck or helo pad will provide excellent anchorage).

Place exercise mats in the center of the ring so that the entire square is filled. Cover the mats with a large sheet of canvas. The canvas may be tucked under the mats, or tacked to a wooden frame placed around the perimeter of the ring. Once the mats are in place, tighten the rope turnbuckles and the guide wire turnbuckles. All ropes should be under tension, and the corner posts firmly anchored.

Two final touches will complete construction of the ring: First, place some foam rubber padding or folded towels around the eyelet bolts on each corner post. This will protect the boxers from possible injury. Finally, swab the mats with a disinfectant solution in order to keep them clear of dirt and debris, and prevent foreign matter from entering a boxer's eyes or open cut.

sport, but it should be well-constructed and built to prevent injury to the participants.

The ring should be 18 by 18 feet, with matting material in the center. At each corner of the square erect a 3-inch-diameter metal post, $4\frac{1}{2}$ feet in length. Weld a 12-by-12-inch steel plate perpendicularly to the bottom of the post. This will keep the post erect. These four corner posts will support the ring ropes. The ropes can be fashioned from wire rope, faced with a smooth rubber hose or

6. Additional Shipboard Physical Fitness Activities

It should be clear by now that the purpose of this book is to convince the reader that physical fitness should be an integral part of shipboard routine. The boxing smoker outlined in Chapter 5 is just one of many ways to combine daily exercise with the enjoyment of recreational activity. There are numerous other shipboard events that can be arranged in an effort to promote morale and involve all hands in some sort of program of physical activity. This final chapter discusses some of these events.

Wrestling smokers are usually quite a bit of fun. There are probably a number of people onboard your ship who have wrestled in college or high school and would enjoy participating or officiating. Some initial planning is required, just as is necessary in presenting a boxing smoker. Conditioning of the participants, proper supervision, and prior planning will all combine to make a wrestling smoker fun for the entire ship's company.

Martial arts have become very popular over the past several years. Many ships have karate and judo clubs that practice onboard at sea, or in the base gym when in port. This is a great way to learn self-defense and to take part in some very vigorous exercise. Take note, of course, that only a qualified instructor should organize such activities, and then only with rigid supervision.

Jogging programs have also gained popularity with sailors, and have met with avid command support. A jogging course may be measured off around the main deck or flight deck. Programs may be designed for distance or time. Group participation in jogging is an outstanding way to promote physical conditioning because the more-experienced members of the group can "pace" the others while those who might be easily discouraged from continuing will be led along by the other members. The command can provide encouragement by awarding printed certificates recognizing a "50-miler club" or "100-miler club," depending on the distance jogged during a deployment period.

Basketball is also a very real possibility on ships at sea. The well deck, hangar bay, or any open area on a weather deck will make a fine basketball court. One-, two-, or three-man basketball can easily be played onboard small ships, and full teams will find sufficient room to play on the larger ships.

Have you ever played volleyball in the middle of the Pacific Ocean? Well, here is how the nuclear guided missile cruiser USS *Long Beach* holds its Sunday afternoon volleyball game.

Start by procuring a suitable court to play in. The flight deck or helo landing pad will suffice. Rig a volleyball net supported by two uprights athwartships, dividing the court into two equal halves. The net should be 7 feet from the deck as measured to the top of the net. Run a length of wire rope along the ship's centerline perpendicular to the net and 10 feet off of the deck. You may secure one end of the wire to a director or gun mount and the other to the stern light or flagstaff. Attach approximately 12 to 15 feet of nylon shot line to a volleyball. (The ship's recreation committee may purchase specially tethered volleyballs, or you can place a standard volleyball in a makeshift mesh net, tying the shot line to the mesh.) Fasten the other end of the shot line to a swivel or small eyelet hook (the one you carry your keys on will do). Clip the swivel hook to the wire rope such that it may slide freely along the entire length of rope. You are now ready to play volleyball without fear of sacrificing the ball to Neptunus Rex!

Exercising in groups is also an interesting possibility (shipboard Marines have been doing this for years). Anyone interested in a group workout at the end of the working day can assemble in an open area for a program of planned exercises. Exercising in a group has several motivating advantages. A group leader can serve to lead the exercises in a planned fashion and at a pace that the group can easily maintain. An individual is also less likely to abandon a physical fitness program if he works out with others to encourage him.

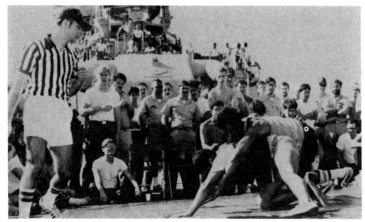

Shipboard Wrestling Smoker

The preceding has presented a few simple ideas offered to promote physical fitness and exercise. The typical sailor's ingenuity, aided by some command support, can result in some very interesting ways to stay fit. An excellent way in which the command can raise the ship's physical fitness consciousness is by establishing a "Captain's Cup" competition. Such a program would call for divisional teams to voluntarily compete against each other in athletic activities. A combination of shipboard and shore activities would balance out the program. Boxing, basketball, wrestling, flag football, bowling, volleyball, golf, soccer, or almost any other sport can be applied to the contest. The winning division would be the one that assembles the greatest number of points from competition. Individual trophies may be awarded for each category, and the overall winning division could receive the "Captain's Cup" and an added privilege, such as a division party or special liberty.

Physical fitness is everyone's responsibility. It is a responsibility that has an important effect on every individual's work, play, and health. Today's shipboard personnel must make a concerted effort to make physical exercise a part of their daily lives, as the unfit person cannot adequately function in the rigorous life at sea. The ever-increasing technical demands associated with the naval service require that the sailor's body and mind function as a finely tuned machine, capable of working hard and effectively.

This book has offered some basic advice on the subject of shipboard physical fitness. Using these basics as a foundation, each and every person who is confined by the space and time limitations of life at sea can keep physically fit and able to enjoy an active, healthy, and productive life.

Notes

1. Robert V. Hockey, *Physical Fitness.* 2nd ed. (St. Louis: C. V. Mosby Co., 1973) p. 12.

2. H. Harrison Clarke, *Application of Measurement to Health and Physical Education.* 4th ed. (Englewood Cliffs, N.J.: Prentice-Hall, 1967) p. 14.

3. Kenneth H. Cooper, *Aerobics.* 3rd ed. (New York: Bantam Books Inc., 1968) p. 13.

4. E. L. Wallis and G. A. Logan, *Figure Improvement and Body Conditioning Through Exercise.* (Englewood Cliffs, N.J.: Prentice-Hall, 1964).

5. Army Times At Your Service Report. "Calorie Check List." (Washington, D.C.: Army Times Publishing Co., 1961).

6. Ibid.